Sacroiliac Joint Pain

Sacroiliac Joint Pain

A Comprehensive Guide to Surgical and Interventional Procedures

EDITED BY

Alaa Abd-Elsayed

AND

Dawood Sayed

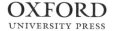

OXFORD
UNIVERSITY PRESS

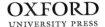

Oxford University Press is a department of the University of Oxford. It furthers
the University's objective of excellence in research, scholarship, and education
by publishing worldwide. Oxford is a registered trade mark of Oxford University
Press in the UK and certain other countries.

Published in the United States of America by Oxford University Press
198 Madison Avenue, New York, NY 10016, United States of America.

Library of Congress Cataloging-in-Publication Data
Names: Abd-Elsayed, Alaa, editor. | Sayed, Dawood, editor.
Title: Sacroiliac joint pain / [edited by] Alaa Abd-Elsayed and Dawood Sayed.
Description: New York, NY : Oxford University Press, [2022] |
Includes bibliographical references and index.
Identifiers: LCCN 2021017659 (print) | LCCN 2021017660 (ebook) |
ISBN 9780197607947 (paperback) | ISBN 9780197607961 (epub) |
ISBN 9780197607978
Subjects: MESH: Sacroiliac Joint | Arthralgia
Classification: LCC RB127.5.C48 (print) | LCC RB127.5.C48 (ebook) |
NLM WE 750 | DDC 616/.0472—dc23
LC record available at https://lccn.loc.gov/2021017659
LC ebook record available at https://lccn.loc.gov/2021017660

DOI: 10.1093/med/9780197607947.001.0001

1 3 5 7 9 8 6 4 2
Printed by Marquis, Canada

To God, my parents, my wife, and my two beautiful kids, Maro and George. To my friend Dr. Sayed for his partnership in editing this book
—Alaa Abd-Elsayed, MD, MPH

I would like to thank my teachers, mentors, family, and friends in their support of me in my endeavor to complete this text. I am greatly thankful to our authors for selflessly volunteering to contribute to this text. To my parents, Jan and Gulnar Sayed, thank you for inspiring me to devote my life to helping others. To my wife, Lindsey, thank you for supporting me and keeping the train on the tracks for our family. To my little girls, Zahra, Farah, and Sabrina, thank you for letting "Dada" spend valuable "playtime" away from you to complete this book. To Dr. Abd-Elsayed, thank you for your partnership and relentlessness to bring this to the finish line. Finally, to God, thank you for all that you have provided me.
—Dawood Sayed, MD

Contents

Part III: Role of regenerative medicine

Part IV: Peripheral nerve stimulation for the sacroiliac joint

Part V: Surgical fusion for the sacroiliac joint

Preface

The sacroiliac joint (SIJ) is one of the major joints in the body that can cause severe chronic pain. Pain caused by the SIJ can significantly impair the ability to perform simple daily activities. Over the years, it has been a focus of research and new therapeutic targets. Management of the SIJ starts with non-pharmacologic modalities like physical therapy, medications, and injections, and if needed proceeds to more advanced interventions such as radiofrequency ablation, neuromodulation, and SIJ fusion. The scope of interventions available for treating SIJ pain has significantly increased over the past decade. We found that there is a significant lack of literature to describe all the advancements in SIJ treatments, which was our inspiration for creating this text.

This book was written by experts in the field of pain management, anesthesiology, physical medicine and rehabilitation, and neurosurgery who shared their expertise in performing different interventions for treating SIJ conditions. This book will serve as a guide to all interventionalists who deal with the SIJ at various levels of training, practice, and specialty. We made every effort to include all the details related to all procedures performed.

We would like to thank all the authors who shared their knowledge writing chapters for this book. We would also like to thank the publisher for sponsoring this book to make it available for practitioners worldwide.

We hope that all readers will enjoy reading this book and that it will guide them to the best practices in interventional management for treating painful SIJ conditions.

Alaa Abd-Elsayed, MD
Dawood Sayed, MD

Contributors

Rany T. Abdallah, MD, PhD, MBA
Medical Director
Department of Pain Management
Center for Interventional Pain and Spine
Milford, DE, USA

Alaa Abd-Elsayed, MD, MPH, FASA
Department of Anesthesiology
University of Wisconsin Hospitals and
  Clinics
University of Wisconsin School
  of Medicine and Public Health
Madison, WI, USA

Gustaf Van Acker, MD, PhD
Instructor
Case Western Reserve University
  School of Medicine
Pain Medicine
MetroHealth Medical System
Cleveland, OH, USA

Haider M. Ali, MD
Resident Physician
Department of Anesthesiology
Ochsner Medical Center
New Orleans, LA, USA

Ajay B. Antony, MD
Interventional Pain
Department of Pain Medicine
The Orthopaedic Institute
Gainesville, FL, USA

Nomen Azeem, MD
Assistant Clinical Professor
Department of Neurology/Pain
University of South Florida
Tampa, FL, USA

Jonathon Belding, MD/MS
Assistant Professor
Case Western Reserve University
  School of Medicine
Department of Orthopedics
Metrohealth Medical System
Cleveland, OH, USA

Nicholas C. Canzanello, DO
Resident Physician
Department of Physical Medicine and
  Rehabilitation
Mayo Clinic
Rochester, MN, USA

Tyler Concannon, MD
Resident Physician
Department of Anesthesiology
University of Kansas Medical Center
Kansas City, KS, USA

Michelle N. Dang, MD
Private Practice
Houston, TX, USA

Yashar Eshraghi, MD
Medical Director, Pain Research
Department of Anesthesia
Interventional Pain Management
Ochsner Health System
New Orleans, LA, USA

Kris Ferguson, MD
Pain Physician
Aspirus Pain Management
Aspirus Hospital
Antigo, WI, USA

Kenneth Fiala, BS
Medical Student
University of Wisconsin-Madison School
    of Medicine and Public Health
Madison, WI, USA

Andrew Frazier, DO
Department of Anesthesiology
The University of Kansas Hospital
Kansas City, KS, USA

Akshat Gargya, MBBS
Assistant Professor
Department of Anesthesiology and
    Pain Management
University of Vermont Medical Center
Burlington, VT, USA

Johnathan Goree, MD
Associate Professor, Director of Chronic
    Pain Division
Department of Anesthesiology
University of Arkansas for Medical Sciences
Little Rock, AR, USA

Maged Guirguis, MD
Associate Professor
Department of Anesthesiology & Critical
    Care Medicine
Ochsner Health System University of
    Queensland Ochsner Medical School
New Orleans, LA, USA

Mayank Gupta, MD
Physician
Kansas Pain Management
Overland Park, KS

Behnum A. Habibi, MD
Assistant Professor
Department of Physical Medicine and
    Rehabilitation
Lewis Katz School of Medicine at Temple
    University
Philadelphia, PA, USA

Jonathan M. Hagedorn, MD
Assistant Professor
Department of Anesthesiology and
    Perioperative Medicine,
    Division of Pain Medicine
Mayo Clinic
Rochester, MN, USA

Benjamin K. Homra, MD
Resident Physician
Department of Anesthesia
Ochsner Clinic Foundation
New Orleans, LA, USA

Hunter Hoopes, OMSIII
Bachelor of Science
Fourth Year Medical Student
Kansas City University
Kansas City, MS, USA

Meghan Cantlon Hughes, MD, MPH
Department of Anesthesiology
University of Wisconsin Hospitals and
    Clinics
University of Wisconsin School of Medicine
    and Public Health
Madison, WI, USA

Christine L. Hunt, DO
Mayo Clinic Minnesota
Division of Pain Medicine
Rochester, MN, USA

Jessica Jameson, MD, FASA
Axis Spine Center
Coeur d'Alene, ID, USA

Navdeep Jassal, MD
Assistant Clinical Professor
Department of Neurology/Pain
University of South Florida
Tampa, FL, USA
Assistant Clinical Professor
Department of Physical Medicine &
    Rehabilitation
University of Central Florida
Orlando, FL, USA
Founder
Spine & Pain Institute of Florida
Lakeland, FL, USA

Mogana V. Jayakumar, DO, MS
Resident Physician
Department of Anesthesiology
New York-Presbyterian Brooklyn
    Methodist Hospital
Brooklyn, NY, USA

Hemant Kalia, MD, MPH, FIPP
Program Director, Interventional Spine &
    Pain Fellowship Program
Physical Medicine & Rehabilitation
Rochester Regional Health System
Rochester, NY, USA

Sarafina Kankam, MD
Interventional Pain Fellow/
    Anesthesiologist
Department of Anesthesiology/
    Chronic Pain Division
University of Arkansas for
    Medical Sciences
Little Rock, AR, USA

Chong H. Kim, MD
Professor
Case Western Reserve University
    School of Medicine
Department of Anesthesiology,
    Department of Physical Medicine
    and Rehabilitation
MetroHealth Medical System
Cleveland, OH, USA

Lisa R. Kroopf, MD
Interventional Pain Physician
CEO Monterey Pain and Spine Institute
Monterey, CA, USA

Usman Latif, MD, MBA
Assistant Professor
Department of Anesthesiology and
    Interventional Pain
The University of Kansas Hospital
Kansas City, KS, USA

Mark N. Malinowski, DO, MS, FIPP
Adena Spine Center
Adena Health System
Chillicothe, OH, USA

Jillian Maloney, MD
Mayo Clinic Arizona
Division of Pain Medicine
Rochester, MN, USA

Joshua Martens, BS
Medical Student
University of Wisconsin-Madison
    School of Medicine and
    Public Health
Madison, WI, USA

Luay Mrad, MD
Fellow
Department of Anesthesiology
    and Pain Management
University of Vermont Medical Center
Burlington, VT, USA

Kemly Philip, MD, PhD, MBE
Resident Physician
Department of Physical Medicine and
    Rehabilitation
McGovern Medical School at
    the University of Texas Health
    Sciences Center
Houston, TX, USA

Dawood Sayed, MD
Professor and Division Chief of Pain
    Medicine
Anesthesiology and Pain Medicine
University of Kansas Medical Center
Kansas City, KS, USA

Samara Shipon, DO
Private Practice
Phoenix, AZ, USA

Gregory Lawson Smith, MD
Assistant Professor
Department of Anesthesiology
University of Arkansas for Medical Sciences
Little Rock, AR, US

Natalie H. Strand, MD
Assistant Professor
Department of Anesthesiology
Mayo Clinic
Phoenix, AZ, USA

Anshuman R. Swain, MD
Attending Physician, President and CEO
Hurricane Pain Management LLC
Columbus, Ohio

Cory Ullger, DO
Pain Medicine Fellow
Department of Pain Medicine/Neurology
University of South Florida
Tampa, FL, USA

Jacqueline Weisbein, DO
Physician
Interventional Pain Management
Napa Valley Orthopaedic Medical Group
Napa, CA, USA

PART I

Sacroiliac joint

Anatomy of the sacroiliac joint

Mark N. Malinowski, Anshuman R. Swain, and
Chong H. Kim

Introduction

The sacroiliac joint (SIJ) is a multiplanar joint located in the dorsal complex of the pelvis.
The SIJ is one of the primary articulations that provides the lower extremities with stability
to enable an erect, stable posture. The SIJ is well endowed with ligaments, owing to the importance of its stability, as it is the primary structure for weight transfer of the trunk to the
pelvis and lower extremities. Furthermore, the joint is well vascularized and heavily innervated, making it a clinically significant structure with respect to primary, autoimmune, and
traumatic disease processes. The chapter will describe the gross anatomy of this joint as well
as its embryologic origins, variability, and proposed movements as it relates to the potential
of the SIJ for pathogenicity.[1]

Gross anatomic and embryologic considerations

The SIJ is the bony articulation of the sacrum and the ipsilateral ilium. This bilateral structure exists in the posterior aspect of the pelvic ring at its anterosuperior end
(Figure 1.1). The superior aspect of the joint approximates the sacral ala anteromedially.
The inferior aspect of the joint approximates the coccyx and sacrococcygeal joint
inferomedially. The inferolateral aspect of the joint approximates the greater sciatic
notch and the piriformis muscle. The entire joint is well encapsulated with ligaments
to be discussed hereafter.[1-4]

The SIJ is considered to be diarthrodial as both osseous ends are covered a thin layer of
cartilage as well as synovium.[1] However, the SIJ has also been classified as amphiarthrodial
because it has a cartilaginous disk-like structure between the bones as well as a syndesmosis.[2-4] Ultimately, the case can be made that it is neither based on the presence of the
interosseous SIJ ligament dorsally,[5] and the abutment within the joint of two different types

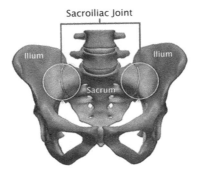

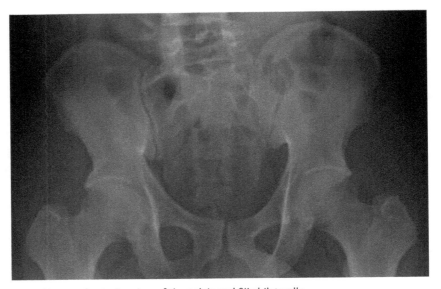

FIGURE 1.1. X-ray and anterior view of the pelvis and SIJs bilaterally.

of cartilage (hyaline [sacrum], fibrocartilage [ilium]) dismisses it as a syndesmosis or symphysis.[1] The auricular shape of the ilium and sacrum is smooth anteriorly, whereas the dorsal aspect is coarse, with varying tuberosities that provide ligamentous attachments (Figure 1.2). The surfaces of the SIJ are flat early in life but become more interdigitated and multifaceted beyond the third decade.[6–8]

The embryologic origin of the SIJ is complex. Mesenchymal cells are oriented into a three-layered structure of cartilage that are dedicated to the sacrum, ilium, and articular cavity. The joint can be identified at a gestational age of 2 months, with cavitation of the joint beginning at the 10th gestational month and extending into adulthood as a result of fibrous cartilage interdigitation within the cavity itself. The sacrum is formed as five independent sacral segments that later fuse to form the triangular bone around age 15 years, but the SIJ is fully apparent and developed at the eighth month of life, and gender-based dimorphism occurs from the eighth gestational month through puberty.[9,10]

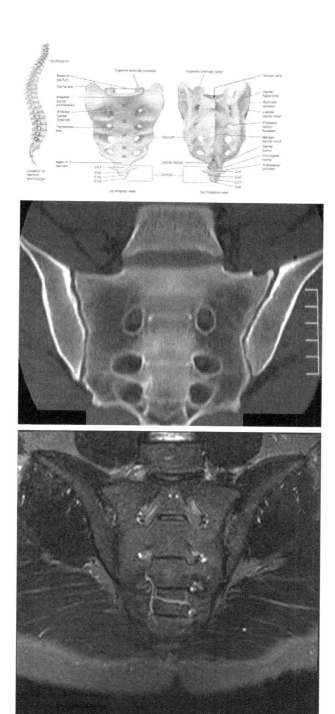

FIGURE 1.2. Computed tomography (CT) and magnetic resonance imaging (MRI) views of the dorsal aspect of the sacrum and its position related to the lumbar spine.

Ligaments of the SIJ

The ligamentous design of the SIJ is robust (Table 1.1).[5] Dorsally, the interosseous sacral ligaments (ISLs) are strong bilateral ligaments that attach to the dorsal sacral tuberosities and fan laterally to solidify the connection of the sacrum to the ilium. These ligaments are oriented dorsolaterally or cranially. Lateral to the interosseous ligament lies the posterior sacroiliac ligaments (PSLs) as they attach the sacrum to the posterior superior iliac spine (PSIS) and nearby bone and, in a similar fashion, run dorsolaterally (cranial group) and cranially (caudal group). Lateral to the PSLs are bilateral sacrospinous ligaments that connect the ischium (ischial spine) to the inferolateral aspect of the sacrum, while the sacrotuberous ligaments (STLs) connect the inferior sacrum to the ischial tuberosities as it coalesces with the PSLs. While not associated with the SIJ, the supraspinous ligament of the lumbar spine becomes confluent with the superficial (and possibly the deep) dorsal sacrococcygeal ligament in the midline as it associates with the sacrococcygeal ligament. Lastly, the iliolumbar ligament (ILL) traverses in a diagonal fashion laterally from the transverse process of the fifth lumbar vertebrae to the anterior or posterior margin of the iliac crest (Figure 1.3). The ILL has a significant amount of variability and may consist of one to four separate bands (dorsal, ventral, lumbosacral and sacroiliac).[5]

The SIJ has a very stable anterior network of ligamentous fibers. The most prominent ligament is the anterior sacroiliac ligament, which forms a strong fibrous capsule as

TABLE 1.1 Ligaments of the SIJ

Ligaments	Anterior/Posterior	Location (From)	Location (To)	Extrinsic/Intrinsic
Anterior sacroiliac ligament (ASL)	Anterior/inferior	Anterior sacrum/ala	Anterior ilium	Intrinsic
Interosseous sacral ligament (ISL)	Posterior	Sacral tuberosity	Iliac tuberosity	Intrinsic
Posterior sacroiliac ligament (PSL)	Posterior	Sacral ala or lateral sacral crest	Ilium or iliac tuberosity	Intrinsic
Long posterior sacroiliac ligament (LPSL)	Posterior	Sacral tubercles	Posterior superior iliac crest	Intrinsic
Iliolumbar ligament (ILL)	Anterior/posterior	Anterior: L5 (or L4) transverse process tip Posterior: L5 transverse process to	Anterior: Iliac crest anterior margin Posterior: Posterior margin of iliac crest	Extrinsic
Sacrotuberous ligament (STL)	Posterior	Caudal edge of sacrum/coccyx	Posterior inferior iliac spine	Extrinsic
Sacrospinous ligament (SSL)	Anterolateral	Anterior S3, S4	Ischial spine	Extrinsic

Adapted from Poilliot et al.[5]

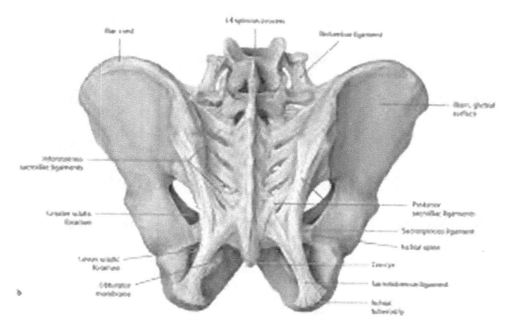

FIGURE 1.3. Posterior aspect of the sacrum and ilium and associated ligamentous structures.

it traverses from medial to lateral in a curvilinear fashion to attach to the ventral aspect of the ilium. The iliolumbar ligament also connects the anterior transverse process of the fifth lumbar vertebra to the corresponding area of the ilium (Figure 1.4).[5]

Muscular structures associated with the SIJ

While there are a variety of muscles that are associated with or are located near the SIJ, there is no clear supporting evidence to suggest that these muscles impact the joint itself. Muscles of the back, pelvis, and lower extremities have some association with the SIJ (Figure 1.5). The erector spinae (ES) muscle group is composed of the iliocostalis, longissimus, and sacrospinalis muscles. This group is known to have some attachment to the SIJ, with the sacrospinalis muscle known to have the preponderance of attachment to the sacrum. The ES group attaches to the lumbar spine and lower thoracic spine as well as the ILL.[11] The multifidus has a strong association with the lumbar spine and, through attachment, is connected to both the ES group and the dorsal sacrum. In addition, there is connectivity with the sacral ligaments, the lumbar spine, and the hip flexors (iliacus, psoas) and pelvic stabilizer muscles (quadratus lumborum). The biceps femoris, semimembranosus, and semitendinosus are muscles of the hamstrings, and there is potential attachment of these muscles with the STL, with the exception of the semitendinosus.[12] Of the muscles of the dorsal pelvis, the gluteus maximus muscles have an extensive attachment to the sacrum

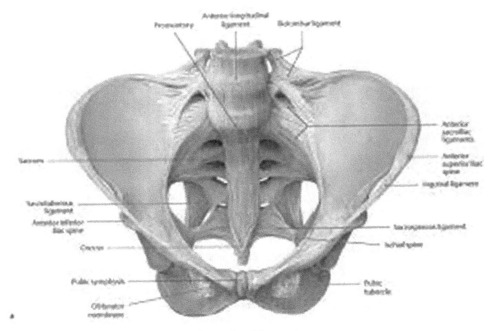

FIGURE 1.4. Ventral aspect of the SIJ and associated ligaments.

and aponeurosis of the ES group, but it is the piriformis muscle that has the most direct attachment to the SIJ. The clinical significance of this attachment is unclear, with no reports of this muscle being involved with movement of this joint.[5]

Innervation and blood supply of the SIJ

The dorsal innervation of the SIJ appears to be better understood than the ventral aspect, as the ventral aspect has been postulated to be supplied by the ventral lumbopelvic rami.[9] The innervation of the SIJ dorsally appears to have wide variability, and this may include myelinated and unmyelinated fibers from both somatic and autonomic sources as the inferior hypogastric plexus traverses ventrally nearby. In a narrative review of the literature, the SIJ appears to be most consistently innervated by the dorsal rami of L5 as well as the dorsal rami of S1 through S3.[9] In some cases, S4 as well as elements from the dorsal root ganglion of L1 through S2 and the superior gluteal and the obturator nerves may also contribute.[13] In fact, both A-delta and C fibers may both extensively innervate the joint as well as surrounding ligaments and joint capsule, as a variety of small-diameter fibers have been found (Figure 1.6).[9,13-15]

The SIJ is endowed with a rich blood supply from branches of the iliac vessels (Figures 1.7 and 1.8). The common iliac artery branches into the external iliac artery (EIA) and the internal iliac artery (IIA). There is some variation of the tributary branches of the EIA and IIA in terms of branching location. The anterior SIJ is primarily supplied by the iliolumbar artery as it branches from the IIA or the common iliac artery. The posterior aspect of the joint is supplied by branches of the superior gluteal artery as it is situated anterior to the

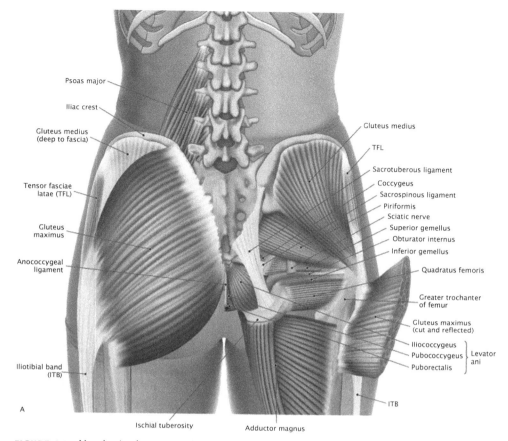

Psoas major

Iliac crest

Gluteus medius
(deep to fascia)

Tensor fasciae
latae (TFL)

Gluteus
maximus

Anococcygeal
ligament

Iliotibial band
(ITB)

A

Ischial tuberosity

Gluteus medius

TFL

Sacrotuberous ligament

Coccygeus

Sacrospinous ligament

Piriformis

Sciatic nerve

Superior gemellus

Obturator internus

Inferior gemellus

Quadratus femoris

Greater trochanter
of femur

Gluteus maximus
(cut and reflected)

Iliococcygeus

Pubococcygeus } Levator
ani

Puborectalis

ITB

Adductor magnus

FIGURE 1.5. Muscles in close approximation with the SIJ.

Muscles of close approximation to the sacroiliac joint; Erector spinae group; Gluteus maximus, medius, minimus; Psoas major, minor; Multifidus; Piriformis; Quadratus lumborum; Biceps femoris; Semimembranosus; Semitendinosus (unclear)

joint. Both the lateral sacral arteries and the median sacral artery perfuse the posterior aspect of the SIJ, arising from the gluteal arteries of the IIA, with the deep, interarticular structures of the SIJ supplied by many penetrating branches.[5] Venous collection is largely dependent on the venous sacral plexus, with continuity with Batson's plexus and ultimately the internal iliac veins (Figure 1.9).[5]

Axes and movement of the SIJ

The intrapelvic axes have been theorized and reviewed to explain the movements of the pelvic bones.[16] The three dimensions of both the sacrum and the ilia and ischia provide a conceptual framework to examine the movements of these bones, and ultimately the SIJ, in both the supine and the upright position (Figure 1.10).[16] The motions of the SIJ have been described as rotation and translation among three axes through a singular point of origin as it relates to an X, Y, and Z Cartesian coordinate system (Figure 1.11).[17,18]

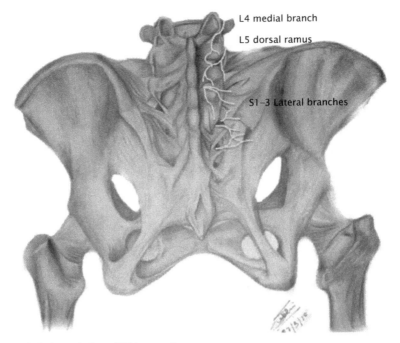

L4 medial branch

L5 dorsal ramus

S1–3 Lateral branches

FIGURE 1.6. Artist's rendering of SIJ innervation.

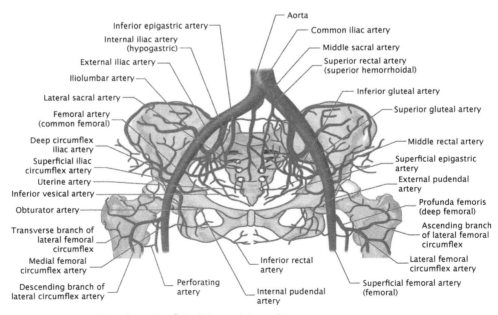

Inferior epigastric artery

Internal iliac artery (hypogastric)

External iliac artery

Iliolumbar artery

Lateral sacral artery

Femoral artery (common femoral)

Deep circumflex iliac artery

Superficial iliac circumflex artery

Uterine artery

Inferior vesical artery

Obturator artery

Transverse branch of lateral femoral circumflex

Medial femoral circumflex artery

Descending branch of lateral circumflex artery

Perforating artery

Aorta

Common iliac artery

Middle sacral artery

Superior rectal artery (superior hemorrhoidal)

Inferior gluteal artery

Superior gluteal artery

Middle rectal artery

Superficial epigastric artery

External pudendal artery

Profunda femoris (deep femoral)

Ascending branch of lateral femoral circumflex

Lateral femoral circumflex artery

Superficial femoral artery (femoral)

Internal pudendal artery

Inferior rectal artery

FIGURE 1.7. Anterior schematic of the SIJ's arterial supply.

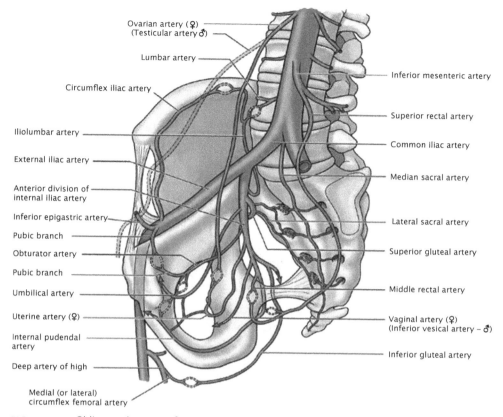

Ovarian artery (♀)
(Testicular artery ♂)

Lumbar artery

Circumflex iliac artery

Iliolumbar artery

External iliac artery

Anterior division of
internal iliac artery

Inferior epigastric artery

Pubic branch

Obturator artery

Pubic branch

Umbilical artery

Uterine artery (♀)

Internal pudendal
artery

Deep artery of high

Medial (or lateral)
circumflex femoral artery

Inferior mesenteric artery

Superior rectal artery

Common iliac artery

Median sacral artery

Lateral sacral artery

Superior gluteal artery

Middle rectal artery

Vaginal artery (♀)
(Inferior vesical artery – ♂)

Inferior gluteal artery

FIGURE 1.8. Oblique schematic of SIJ's arterial supply as it relates to the internal and external iliac arteries.

The most significant and practical analysis of the movement of the SIJ is the position and motion that occurs in the upright and standing position. The transfer of forces is bidirectional, with downward pressure of the torso to the pelvis and corresponding upward pressure of the lower extremities, and thus pelvic bones, to maintain this upright position. These forces are appropriately opposed by the rigorous ligamentous architecture encapsulating the SIJ complex, and they are at significant juxtaposition to both maintain healthy biomechanics and be subject to pathologic disposition. The most accepted concept of movement under these circumstances is the ventral displacement of the sacral ala by downward truncal pressure coupled with the dorsal displacement and rotation of the Ilium by cephalad force of the femurs. The motion of the sacrum in this position is nutation around the transverse axis through the level of the S2 neuroforamen and exaggerates the lumbar lordosis. The opposite movement, counternutation, occurs to reduce the lumbar lordosis, and this movement is suggested to be between 3 and 6 mm.[9]

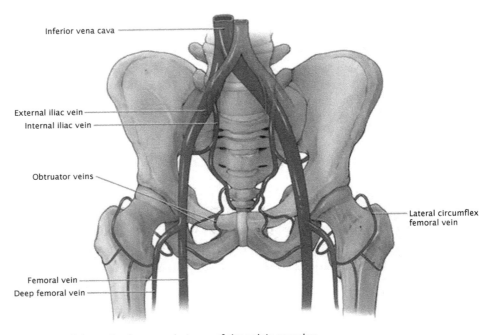

FIGURE 1.9. Schematic of venous drainage of the pelvic complex.

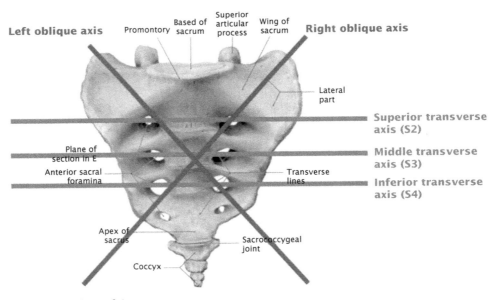

FIGURE 1.10. Axes of the sacrum.

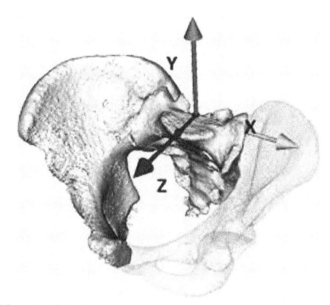

FIGURE 1.11. Schematic of the Cartesian coordinate system as it relates to the SIJ.

Anatomic variations of the SIJ

Lumbosacral transitional anatomy is a common finding in clinical practice. The presence of anatomic variants to the "traditional" anatomy poses a unique problem in clinical practice in an already elusive pain generator.[19,20] In a study of 534 patients undergoing computed tomography of the pelvis, six types of anatomic variants were noted.[3] Accessory SIJs represented the most common variant (19.1% of the sampled scans) and had a higher incidence in patients who were obese, of advanced age, and male. Together with transitional anatomy, these variations in the morphology require additional consideration in the clinical setting of back pain and interventional care when these radiographic findings are present.

References

1. Wong M, Sinkler MA, Kiel J. Anatomy, Abdomen and Pelvis, Sacroiliac Joint. In: StatPearls. StatPearls Publishing, Treasure Island (FL); 2020.
2. Postacchini R, Trasimeni G, Pipani F, Sessa P, Perotti S, Postacchini F. Morphometric anatomical and CT study of the human adult sacroiliac region. Surg Radiol Anat 2017; 39: 85–94.
3. Prassopoulos P, Panos K, Faflia C, Voloudaki A, Gourtsoyiannis N. Sacroiliac joints: Anatomical variants on CT. J Comp Tomogr 1999; 23(2): 323–327.
4. Gerlach U, Lierse W. Functional construction of the sacroiliac ligamentous apparatus. Acta Anat 1992; 144: 97–102.
5. Poilliot A, Zwirner J, Doyle T, Hammer N. A systematic review of the normal sacroiliac joint anatomy and adjacent tissues for pain physicians. Pain Physician 2019; 22: E247–E274.
6. Nishi K, Tsurumoto T, Okamoto K, Ogami-Takamura K, Hasegawa T, Moriuchi T, Sakamoto J, Oyamada J, Higashi T, Manabe Y, Saiki K. Three-dimensional morphological analysis of the human sacroiliac joint: Influences on the degenerative changes of the auricular surfaces. J Anat 2018; 232: 238–249.

7. Rosatelli A, Agur A, Chhaya S. Anatomy of the interosseous region of the sacroiliac joint. J Orthop Sports Phys Ther 2006; 36(4): 200–208.

8. Walker J. Ager-related differences in the human sacroiliac joint: A histological study; implications for therapy. J Orthop Sports Phys Ther 1986; 7(6): 325–334.

9. Vleeming A, Schuenke M, Masi A, Carreiro J, Danneels L, Willard F. The sacroiliac joint: An overview of its anatomy, function and potential for clinical implications. J Anat 2012; 221: 537–567.

10. Krmek N, Jo-Osvatic A, Nikolic T, Krmek V, Salamon A. Anthropological measurement of the sacroiliac joint. Coll Antropol 2006; 30(4): 811–814.

11. McGrath C, Nicholson H, Hurst P. The long posterior sacroiliac ligament: A histological study of morphological relations in the posterior sacroiliac region. Joint Bone Spine 2009; 76(1): 57–62.

12. Fortin J, Kissling R, O'Connor B, Vilensky J. Sacroiliac joint innervation and pain. Am J Orthop 1999; 28: 687–690.

13. Arab A, Nourbakhsh M, Mohammadifar A. The relationship between hamstring length and gluteal muscle strength in individuals with sacroiliac joint dysfunction. J Manual Manip Ther 2011; 19(1): 5–10.

14. Simopoulos T, Manchikanti L, Singh V, Gupta S, Hameed H, Diwan S, Cohen S. A systematic evaluation of the prevalence and diagnostic accuracy of sacroiliac joint interventions. Pain Physician 2012; 15: E305–E344.

15. Cohen S. Sacroiliac joint pain: A comprehensive review of anatomy, diagnosis and treatment. Anesth Analg 2005; 101: 1440–1453.

16. Alderink G. The sacroiliac joint: Review of anatomy, mechanics and function. J Orthop Sports Phys Ther 1991; 13(2): 71–84.

17. Smidt G, McQuade K, Wei S, Barakatt E. Sacroiliac kinematics for reciprocal straddle positions. Spine 1999; 20(9): 1047–1054.

18. McGrath Goode A, Hegedus E, Sizer P, Brismee J, Linberg A, Cook C. Three-dimensional movements of the sacroiliac joint: A systematic review of the literature and assessment of clinical utility. J Manual Manip Ther 2008; 16(1): 25–38.

19. Vanelderen P, Szadek K, Cohen S, De Witte J, Lataster A, Patijn J, Mekhail N, van Kleef M, Zundert J. Sacroiliac joint pain. Pain Practice 2010; 10(5): 470–478.

20. Mahato N. Asymmetric sacroiliac joint anatomy in partial lumbosacral transitional variations: Potential impact on clinical testing in sacral dysfunctions. Med Hypotheses 2019; 124: 110–113.

2

Sacroiliac joint conditions

Anshuman R. Swain, Chong H. Kim, and
Mark N. Malinowski

Multiple pathologic and nonpathologic conditions can result in sacroiliac joint (SIJ) pain (Box 2.1). These conditions can be divided into two general categories: intraarticular (e.g., infection, arthritis, spondyloarthropathies, and malignancy) and extraarticular (e.g., enthesopathy, fracture, ligamentous injuries, and myofascial conditions).[1-3]

Osteoarthritis

Osteoarthritis of the SIJ is the third most common cause of chronic low back pain and is present in 13% to 18.5% of all chronic low back pain patients.[4,5] Degenerative changes of the SIJ may begin at an early age, and they initially affect the iliac cartilage to a greater extent than the sacral cartilage. The reason that the iliac cartilage is affected initially and more significantly is that perpendicular load significantly reduces the extent of degeneration of the sacral articular cartilage but results in additional shearing forces on the iliac articular surface. The result is accelerated degenerative changes, which may present as early as puberty. The sacral articular cartilage generally remains unaltered until advanced age.[4,6] Aside from mechanical differences, the sacral cartilage and the iliac cartilage differ morphologically: The sacral cartilage is rich with acidic-like aminoglycans and is two to three times thicker than the fibrocartilaginous structure of the iliac cartilage.[4,6]

SIJ dysfunction

SIJ dysfunction is a type of nonspecific low back pain; nonspecific low back pain accounts for 85% of acute low back pain syndromes.[7-10] SIJ dysfunction and pain represents a syndrome caused by a combination of pelvic rotation, joint locking, hyper/hypomobility, and/or muscular imbalance.[7] There are no consistent radiographic joint abnormalities, and the

---

BOX 2.1. Causes of SIJ pain

Intraarticular pain
    Osteoarthritis
    Sacroiliac joint dysfunction
    Spondyloarthropathy
    Malignancy
    Trauma
    Infection

Extraarticular pain
    Osteoarthritis
    Sacroiliac joint dysfunction
    Ligamentous injury
    Trauma
    Malignancy
    Myofascial pain
    Enthesopathy
    Pregnancy

From references 2 and 3.

---

diagnosis is often made by physical examination. Physical examination includes pelvic alignment and mobility tests as well as provocative maneuvers that stress the SIJ, attempting to reproduce the patient's pain complaint.[7]

Direct muscular activity cannot cause movement of the SIJ but can place the joint under strain indirectly, resulting in maintenance of a rotated position by a group of muscles acting through the pubic ring. Patients use their hip girdle to stabilize the lumbosacral spine.[7] There are several patterns of SIJ malalignment and muscular dysfunction. The most common pattern of dysfunction involves right anterior and left posterior innominate rotation with sacral torsion ("innominate" refers to the iliac bone).[7]

Infection

SIJ infection is an uncommon spinal infection and is most common in children and young adults; it less frequently affects older patients.[11] SIJ infection can be either pyogenic or granulomatous and is most often unilateral (Figure 2.1). There are a number of predisposing conditions, including drug abuse and intraarticular steroid injection, but nearly 50% of cases present without predisposing factors that can be identified.[12] The pathophysiology of SIJ infection is thought to be hematogenous spread of bacteria from a distant source of

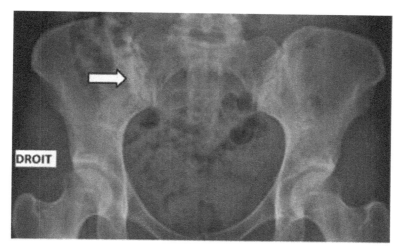

FIGURE 2.1. Infectious sacroiliitis: widening of the left SIJ secondary to infectious process (*white arrow*).[15]

infection to the SIJ, but positive blood cultures have been demonstrated in less than 25% of previously reported cases, and in up to 40% of cases no primary infectious source could be identified.[11–16]

Pyogenic sacroiliitis is the most frequently reported type of SIJ infection. It is most frequently a disease of young adults between the ages of 20 and 30 but has been identified in patients aged 1 to 72 years.[14,15] The infection is typically unilateral in the patient experiences a fever with continuous pain originating in the affected SIJ, with symptoms most prevalent in the buttock, low back, and hip area. Occasionally, pain can radiate to the lower leg. Acute abdominal pain, most frequently in the lower quadrants as well as pain on rectal examination, has been reported in approximately 10% of patients with pyogenic sacroiliitis.[16,17] Severe cases may present with a patient who cannot move in bed with an extended and externally rotated leg or flexed at the hip and abducted. These leg positions are the result of spasm of the proximal piriformis muscle.[16] Patients frequently present with a limp and the inability to bear weight on the ipsilateral leg. Sacroiliac tenderness is a consistent finding on physical examination, and maneuvers that stress the SIJ may trigger excruciating pain. Passive range of motion of the hip joint is usually unlimited and often rules out acute hip joint disease.[14]

Laboratory evaluation demonstrates elevations in the erythrocyte sedimentation rate (ESR) and C-reactive protein (CRP) levels, but leukocytosis is less common.[14,16] Blood cultures can be negative in up to 50% of patients with pyogenic sacroiliitis, particularly in the pediatric population.[18] Imaging-guided SIJ aspiration should be performed in patients if the clinician has high clinical suspicion for pyogenic sacroiliitis and if blood cultures are negative, particularly if the patient is not responding well to empiric antibiotic therapy.[14]

The most common pathogens reported in pyogenic sacroiliitis are *Staphylococcus aureus* and *Pseudomonas aeruginosa*. Empiric antibiotic therapy should always be directed against *S. aureus* and gram-negative organisms, including *P. aeruginosa*. Antimicrobial therapy should be continued for at least 4 to 8 weeks and should be guided by the patient status, pathogen, and presence of complications.[14]

Brucella can cause both septic and reactive sacroiliitis. The SIJ is the most frequently reported location of brucellosis and is seen in more than 10% of patients.[14,18–20] Brucella sacroiliitis has been described as a relatively mild disease with a good prognosis.[21] In rare cases brucellosis may manifest with acute sacroiliitis that has a similar clinical presentation to pyogenic sacroiliitis.[22] While unilateral involvement is more common, bilateral involvement of the SIJ can be seen in up to 25% of patients, particularly those with concurrent spondylitis and peripheral arthritis.[20] The history often includes intake of unpasteurized dairy products as well as clinical signs such as fever, sweating, malaise, and hepatosplenomegaly. In patients suspected of having brucellosis, a Rose bengal test should be performed, particularly if the clinical picture includes septic sacroiliitis and negative blood cultures. Patients usually respond well to treatment with doxycycline and rifampicin.[19]

Crystalline-induced sacroiliitis

The SIJ can be affected by crystal deposition found in gout and calcium pyrophosphate dihydrate (CPPD) deposition disease.[23] Gouty sacroiliitis is typically asymptomatic. Most reported patients have been postmenopausal women with a previous history of gout and acute onset of sacroiliac pain. The patient may present with a fever, and the ESR and CRP levels are frequently elevated in acute gouty sacroiliitis. Physical examination that reveals gouty tophi and elevated uric acid levels should raise suspicion for gouty sacroiliitis in the appropriate clinical setting. Pyogenic sacroiliitis should also be considered in the patient with a history of gout, and diagnostic aspiration of the involved SIJ may provide a definitive diagnosis. The examination of the SIJ aspirate should include polarized microscopy. There has been reports of gouty involvement of the SIJ without any advanced gouty peripheral arthritis or visible tophi.[24] CPPD deposition disease can result in asymptomatic chondrocalcinosis of the SIJ in up to 40% of patients.[25] Diagnosis is made based on the clinical picture of aseptic sacroiliitis, linear calcific deposits within the affected SIJ, and polyarticular chondrocalcinosis.[26] Crystalline-induced sacroiliitis can respond to treatment with nonsteroidal anti-inflammatory drugs (NSAIDs), colchicine, and corticosteroids. Corticosteroids can be administered systemically or by SIJ injection.[24,26]

Spondyloarthropathies

Axial spondyloarthritis is an inflammatory arthritis of the SIJ and the spine.[27,28] The most common adult seronegative spondyloarthropathies are ankylosing spondylitis, reactive arthritis (previously known as Reiter syndrome), and psoriatic arthropathy. Ankylosing spondylitis and reactive arthritis will be discussed in further detail due to the higher incidence of sacroiliac involvement compared to psoriatic arthropathy (Table 2.1).

The most characteristic feature of ankylosing spondylitis is new bone formation resulting in ankylosis of the SIJ and syndesmophyte formation in the spine (Figure 2.2).[28]

TABLE 2.1 Adult seronegative spondyloarthopathies with the most SIJ involvement

Characteristic	Ankylosing spondylitis	Reactive arthritis (Reiter syndrome)	Psoriatic arthropathy
HLA-B27 positive	90%	60–80%	50%
Sacroiliitis	Almost 100%	<50%	20%
Symmetry of sacroiliitis	Symmetric	Asymmetric	Asymmetric
Onset	Gradual	Acute	Variable
Ocular symptoms	30%	Common	Occasional
Gender ratio	Males 3 times more likely	Primarily males	Equal
Peripheral joint involvement	25%	90%	>90%

From reference 29.

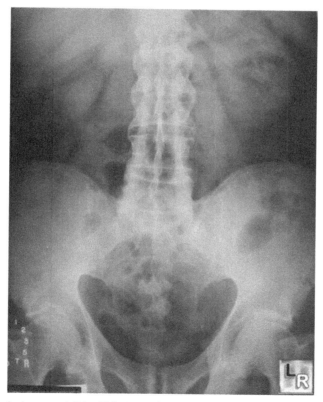

FIGURE 2.2. Ankylosing spondylitis: SIJ fusion with spinal syndesmophyte formation.[32]

Bone formation contributes to disease burden independent of pain and stiffness, eventually resulting in loss of joint space due to cartilage loss, which is followed by cartilaginous fusion and then bony fusion.

A key component to spondyloarthropathies is the development of enthesopathy, which is defined as inflammation at the insertion of tendons, ligaments, or the capsule of the joint.[28] The anatomy of the SIJ can be divided into two areas: the SIJ and the supraarticular zone. Ankylosis of the SIJ area begins within the joint space and then extends into the supraarticular zone and involves the supraarticular ligament.[29,30] The sacroiliac area passes through three stages in the development of ankylosing spondylitis: (1) development of and situs of the joint space; (2) lysis followed by sclerosis; and (3) bony ankylosis, which reflects a reparative ossification.[31]

Reactive arthritis

Reactive arthritis is a spondyloarthropathy that frequently afflicts the SIJ. This condition was previously known as Reiter syndrome,[32–39] but the name has been changed to reactive arthritis because of the namesake's participation in Nazi medical experimentation.[36] The condition refers to an infection-induced systemic illness with sterile synovitis occurring in a genetically predisposed individual secondary to a bacterial infection of the genitourinary (GU) or gastrointestinal (GI) system.[37,38] Reactive arthritis is more frequently reported in males under the age of 40.[39] Multiple GU/GI pathogens can trigger reactive arthritis. The bacteria may reach the afflicted joint in a fragmented or complete form.[39] All triggering pathogens are intracellular organisms; *Chlamydia trachomatis* is the most common GU pathogen and *Salmonella enterica* is the most common GI pathogen reported.[39]

Reactive arthritis presents as a peripheral monoarthritis or an asymptomatic oligoarthritis, enthesitis, or dactylitis (Figure 2.3). Musculoskeletal symptoms present days to several weeks after the inciting infection has occurred. Often, symptoms of the inciting infection have completely resolved by the time musculoskeletal signs and symptoms present.[40] Reactive arthritis typically occurs in the lower extremities; involvement of the axial skeleton is less common. The syndrome may affect the SIJs, the lumbar spine, and less commonly the thoracic or cervical spine. Low back pain is a very common symptom. Warmth and joint effusion may be present over the afflicted joint. Joint involvement may be sequential rather than simultaneous.[40]

Treatment is begun with NSAIDs to reduce the development of syndesmophytes and for analgesic effects. Disease-modifying antirheumatic drugs (DMARDs) are effective for peripheral joint involvement but are not as effective if there is axial joint involvement.[39]

Malignancy

Both primary and secondary malignancies of the sacrum and SIJ can result in SIJ pain. However, the sacrum is four times less likely than the remainder of the spinal column to be

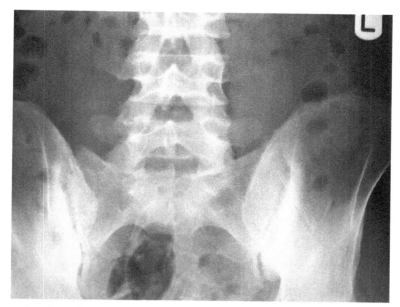

FIGURE 2.3. Reactive arthritis: bilateral, asymmetric sacroiliitis.[15]

the source of a primary bone malignancy.[41,42] Furthermore, the sacrum can be the site for both benign and malignant bone lesions.

Hemangioma is the most commonly identified angiomatous lesion of bone and soft tissue.[43] The sacrum is the site of less than 1% of all osseous hemangiomas.[42,44] Most sacral lesions are asymptomatic and are found incidentally.[42]

Osteoid osteoma is a common benign lesion that involves the spine in 10% of cases, 2% of which are in the sacrum. Patients frequently present with back pain and demonstrate a 2–3:1 male predominance.[45] Pain is usually worst at night and is relieved with NSAIDs. There may be associated muscle atrophy, radicular symptoms, and scoliosis.

Osteoblastoma accounts for 1% of primary bone tumors and has been described in nearly every bone in the human skeleton.[46,47] Up to 45% of cases present in the spine, with the sacrum being the least likely site. Posterior elements are frequently involved, and the lesion may extend into the vertebral body. Sacral lesions are often larger at presentation, likely due to the longer period of symptoms before detection.[42]

Giant cell tumor involves the spine in 7% of all cases and accounts for up to 15% of all lesions of the spine (excluding myeloma). The majority of giant cell tumors arise in the sacrum, and these lesions represent 71% of benign sacral tumors.[48,49] Giant cell tumor is the second most common primary osseous tumor of the sacrum. These lesions present in an eccentric location and in the upper sacrum. Lesions in the sacrum may invade the SIJ.[50,51] Patients frequently present in the third or fourth decade of life. Women are more frequently affected, and pain presents in a nonspecific pattern. Radicular symptoms can be present in up to 33% of cases. Pregnancy-related hormonal

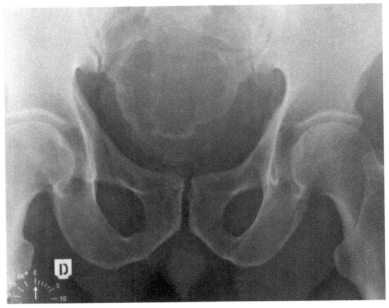

FIGURE 2.4. Chordoma: plain radiograph of the pelvis showing expansion of the sacrum, bone rarefaction, and large mass of soft tissue with some trabeculations.[15]

stimulation may result in dramatic increase in lesion size.[42] Giant cell tumors of the spine are difficult to resect and are more likely to recur than most benign spine lesions; recurrence rates have been reported to be as high as 40% to 60%. Unresectable lesions are treated by radiation therapy or embolization. Lesions invading the SIJ are often considered unresectable.[42]

Chordoma is the most common primary nonlymphoproliferative malignant bone tumor of the spine (Figure 2.4). The sacrococcygeal area represents the most frequent site of this lesion, with up to 60% of all chordomas presenting in the sacrum and coccyx (Figure 2.5).[52,53] Lesions present insidiously due to the slow-growing nature of this tumor, with varying amounts of neurologic involvement depending on the lesion level. Sacral lesions present with motor and sensory disturbances, change in bowel habits, and incontinence.[54] Prognosis of this lesion is dependent on complete resection, which may be difficult because these lesions are often large at presentation and are situated in surgically challenging locations

Ewing tumor is the most common nonlymphoproliferative primary malignant osseous tumor of the spine in children.[42,55,56] It most commonly affects the sacrum.[54] The tumor is typically central in the vertebral body, with extension into the posterior elements seen frequently. Chemotherapy and radiation treatment have significantly improved survivability in patients with Ewing tumor.[57,58] Prognosis is dependent on tumor location. Patients with nonsacral lesions experience nearly 100% local control and 86% of patients have long-term survival. Unfortunately, patients with sacral involvement frequently have a poor prognosis because the lesions are larger at initial presentation.[58]

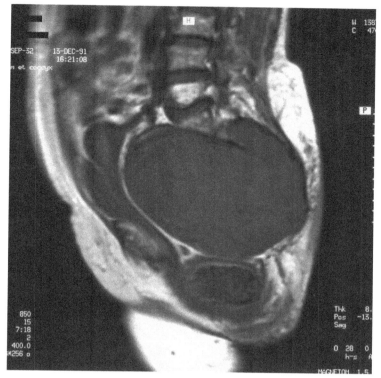

FIGURE 2.5. Sacrococcygeal chordoma.[15]

Trauma

Trauma resulting in pelvic ring injuries may result in SIJ injury. SIJ injury may be the result of repetitive microtrauma or acute trauma. Pelvic ring injuries can be separated into three categories: anterior-posterior compression, lateral compression, and vertical shear injuries.[59] The SIJ may be injured via incomplete sacroiliac dislocation, complete sacroiliac dislocation, or sacroiliac fracture–dislocation.[59]

There are also three major fracture classifications that affect the SIJ:

- A type I fracture involves the anterior aspect of the S2 foramen and results in a large crescent-shaped fragment that is stable. This type of fracture is often minor and less than one-third of the SIJ is involved. A type I fracture involves the least amount of ligamentous injury of the three types of sacroiliac fracture described.
- A type II fracture occurs between the anterior aspect of the S1 and S2 foramen and results in a smaller crescent-shaped fragment compared to a type I injury. A type II fracture occurs when up to two-thirds of the SIJ is involved.
- A type III fracture involves the superior and posterior aspects of the SIJ up to the S1 nerve root. Greater than two-thirds of the SIJ is affected and there is a higher degree of ligamentous injury. A type III fracture is usually smaller than a type I or type II fracture.

Posterior fracture–dislocations of the SIJ involve variable damage to the sacroiliac ligament complex.[59-61]

Pregnancy

The pregnant patient may develop low back pain related to SIJ dysfunction. Many of the joints of the pelvis become more relaxed during pregnancy. During pregnancy, the hormone relaxin causes joint mobility and the pelvis widens, resulting in increased SIJ mobility.[59] The expectant patient may experience SIJ pain as the hips rotate, resulting in increased stress on the SIJ. Pain may be unilateral or bilateral.[62,63] SIJ pain during pregnancy is a component of pelvic girdle pain. Patients with pelvic girdle pain during pregnancy often have higher rates of disability in comparison to patients suffering mechanical low back pain. Risk factors for SIJ dysfunction during pregnancy include forceps delivery, intense contractions, and fetal macrosomia. Minor factors include multiparty, precipitous labor, and a rapid second stage of labor.

References

1. Vanelderen P, Szadek K, Cohen SP, et al. Sacroiliac joint pain. *J Pain Pract.* 2010; 10(5): 470–478.
2. Kiapour A, Joukar A, Elgafy H, et al. Biomechanics of the sacroiliac joint: Anatomy, function, biomechanics, sexual dimorphism, and causes of pain. *Int J Spine Surg.* 2020; 14(suppl. 1): S3–13.
3. Holmes SL, Cohen SP, Cullen MFL, et al. Sacroiliac joint pain. In Binit J. Shah and Mehul J. Desai (Eds.), *Pain medicine: An interdisciplinary case-based approach* (pp. 160–182). Oxford University Press, 2015.
4. Laplante BL, DePalma MJ. Spine osteoarthritis. *PM R.* 2012; 4(5 Suppl): S28–S36.
5. DePalma M, Ketchum J, Queler E, et al. What is the etiology of low back pain, and does age effect the prevalence of each etiology? An interim analysis of 170 consecutive cases. *Pain Med.* 2009; 10: 949.
6. Kampen WU, Tillman B. Age-related changes in the articular cartilage of the human sacroiliac joint. *Anat Embryol.* 1998; 198: 505–551.
7. Clavel A. Sacroiliac joint dysfunction: From a simple pain in the butt to integrated care for complex low back pain. *Tech Reg Anesth Pain Manag.* 2011; 15: 40–50.
8. Deyo RA, Mirza SK, Martin BI. Back pain prevalence and visit rates: Estimates from U.S. national surveys. *Spine.* 2006; 31(23): 2724–2727.
9. Fritz JM, Cleland JA, Childs JD. Subgrouping patients with low back pain: Evolution of a classification approach to physical therapy. *J Orthop Sports Phys Ther.* 2007; 37: 290–302.
10. Jarvik JG, Deyo RA. Diagnostic evaluation of low back pain with emphasis on imaging. *Ann Intern Med.* 2002; 32: 1430–1434.
11. Zimmermann III, B, Mikolich DJ, Lally EV. Septic sacroiliitis. *Sem Arthritis Rheum.* 1996: 26(3): 592–604.
12. Groves C, Cassar-Pullicino V. Imaging of bacterial infections of the sacroiliac joint. *Radiologe.* 2004; 44(3): 242–253.
13. Vyskocil JJ, McIlroy MA, Brennan TA, Wilson FM. Pyogenic infection of the sacroiliac joint: Case reports and review of the literature. *Medicine.* 1991; 70: 188–197.
14. Slobodin G, Rimar D, Boulman N, et al. Acute sacroiliitis. *Clin Rheumatol.* 2016; 35: 851–856.
15. Medscape. Septic Sacroiliitis: The Overlooked Diagnosis. May 01, 2001.
16. Doita M, Yoshiya S, Nabeshima Y, et al. Acute pyogenic sacroiliitis without predisposing conditions. *Spine.* 1976; 28(18): E384–E389.
17. Carlson SA, Jones JS. Pyogenic sacroiliitis. *Am J Emerg Med.* 1994; 12(6): 639–641.
18. Cohn SM, Schoetz DJ Jr. Pyogenic sacroiliitis: Another initiator of the acute abdomen. *Surgery.* 1986; 100(1): 95–98.

19. Wu MS, Chang SS, Lee SH, et al. Pyogenic sacroiliitis—a comparison between pediatric and adult patients. *Rheumatology*. 2007; 46(11): 1684–1687.

20. Ariza J, Pujol M, Valverde, J, et al. Brucellar sacroiliitis: Findings in 63 episodes and current relevance. *Clin Infect Dis*. 1993; 16(6): 761–765.

21. Geyik MF, Gur A, Nas K, et al. Musculoskeletal involvement of brucellosis in different age groups: A study of 195 cases. *Swiss Med Weekly*. 2002; 132 (7–8): 98–105.

22. Dayan L, Deyev S, Palma L, Rozen N. Long-standing, neglected sacroiliitis with marked sacroiliac degenerative changes as a result of Brucella spp. infection. *Spine J*. 2009; 9(3): e1–e4.

23. Ozgul A, Yazicioglu K, Gunduz S, et al. Acute Brucella sacroiliitis: Clinical features. *Clin Rheumatol*. 1998; 17 (6): 521–523.

24. Konatalapalli RM, Demarco PJ, Jelinek JS, et al. Gout in the axial skeleton. *J Rheumatol*. 2009; 36(3): 609–613.

25. Bastani B, Vermuri R, Gennis M. Acute gouty sacroiliitis: A case report and review of the literature. *Mt. Sinai J Med*. 1997; 64(6): 383–385.

26. El Maghraoui A, Lecoules S, Lechevalier D, et al. Acute sacroiliitis as a manifestation of calcium pyrophosphate dihydrate crystal deposition disease. *Clin Exp Rheumatol*. 1999; 17(4): 477–478.

27. Francois S, Guaydier-Souquieres G, Marcelli C. Acute sacroiliitis as a manifestation of calcium pyrophosphate dihydrate crystal deposition disease. A report of two cases. *Rev Rheum Engl Ed*. 1997; 64(7–9): 508–512.

28. De Konig A, Schoones JW, van der Heijde D, van Gaalen FA. Pathophysiology of axial spondylosis arthritis: Consensus and controversies. *Eur J Clin Invest*. 2018; 48: E12913.

29. Dreyfuss P, Dreyer SJ, Cole A, Mayo K. Sacroiliac joint pain. *J Am Acad Orthop Surg*. 2004; 12(4): 255–265.

30. Landewe R, Dougados M, Mielants H, et al. Physical function in ankylosing spondylitis is independently determined by both disease activity and radiographic damage of the spine. *Ann Rheum Dis*. 2009; 68: 863–867.

31. Bleil J, Maier R, Hempfing A, et al. Histomorphologic and histomorphometric characteristics of zygapophyseal joint remodeling in ankylosing spondylitis. *Arthritis Rheumatol*. 2014; 66:1745–1754.

32. http://learningradiology.com/archives05/COW%20134-Ankylosing%20Spondylitis/ankspondylocorrect.htm

33. Fournie B. Pathology and clinic-pathologic correlations in spondyloarthropathies. *Joint Bone Spine*. 2004; 71(6): 525–529.

34. Forestier J. The importance of sacro-iliac change in the early diagnosis of ankylosing spondylarthritis. *Radiology*. 1939; 33: 389–402.

35. Keynan Y, Rimar D. Reactive arthritis—the appropriate name. *Isr Med Assoc J*. 2008; 10(4): 256–258.

36. Panush R, Wallace D, Dorff R, Engleman E. Retraction of the suggestion to use the term "Reiter's syndrome" sixty-five years later. *Arthritis Rheum*. 2007; 56(2): 693–694.

37. Stavropoulos P, Soura E, Kanelleas A, et al. Reactive arthritis. *J Eur Acad Dermatol Venereol* . 2015; 29(3): 415–424.

38. Hannu T. Reactive arthritis. *Best Pract Res Clin Rheumatol*. 2011; 25(3): 347–357.

39. Garcia-Kutzbach A, Chacon-Suchite J, Garcia-Ferrer H, Iraheta I. Reactive arthritis: Update 2018. *Clin Rheumatol*. 2018; 37:869–874.

40. Schmitt SK. Reactive arthritis. *Infect Dis Clin North Am*. 2017; 31: 265–277.

41. Carter J, Hudson A. Reactive arthritis: Clinical aspects and medical management. *Rheum Dis Clin North Am*. 2009; 35(1): 21–44.

42. Fleming DJ, Murphey MD, Carmichael BB, Bernard SA. Primary tumors of the spine. *Semin Musculoskelet Radiol*. 2000; 4(3): 299–320.

43. Murphey MD, Fairbairn KJ, Parman LM, et al. From the archives of the AFIP. Musculoskeletal angiomatous lesions: Radiologic pathologic correlation. *Radiographics*. 1995; 15: 893–917.

44. Mirra JM. Vascular tumors. In JM Mirra (Ed.), *Bone tumors: Clinical, radiologic, and pathologic considerations* (pp. 1340–1478). Lea & Febiger, 1989.

45. Kransdorf MJ, Stull MA, Gilkey GW, Moser RP Jr. Osteoid osteoma. *Radiographics*. 1991; 11:671–696.

46. Seider MJ, Rich TA, Ayala AG, Murray JA. Giant cell tumors of bone: Treatment with radiation therapy. *Radiology*. 1986; 161:537–540.

47. Greenspan A. Benign bone-forming lesions: Osteoma, osteoid osteoma, and osteoblastoma: Clinical, imaging, pathologic, and differential considerations. *Skeletal Radiol*. 1993; 22: 457–459.

48. Shaikh MI, Saifuddin A, Natali C, et al. Spinal osteoblastoma: CT and MR imaging with pathologic correlation. *Skeletal Radiol*. 1999; 28: 33–40.

49. Sanjay BKS, Sim FH, Unni KK, et al. Giant cell tumors of the spine. *J Bone Joint Surg [Br]*. 1993; 75: 148–154.

50. Disler DG, Miklic D. Imaging findings in tumors of the sacrum. *AJR Am J Roentgenol*. 1999; 173: 1699–1706.

51. Eckardt JJ, Grogan TJ. Giant cell tumor of bone. *Clin Orthop*. 1986; 204: 45–58.

52. Smith J, Wixson D, Watson RC. Giant-cell tumor of the sacrum: Clinical and radiologic features in 13 patients. *J Can Assoc Radiol*. 1974; 303: 34–39.

53. Meyer JE, Lepke RA, Lindfors KK, et al. Chordomas: Their CT appearance in the cervical, thoracic, and lumbar spine. *Radiology*. 1984; 153: 693–696.

54. Healey JH, Lane JM. Chordoma: A critical review of diagnosis and treatment. *Orthop Clin North Am*. 1989; 20: 417–426.

55. York JE, Kaczaraj A, Abi-Said D, et al. Sacral chordoma: 40 year experience at a major cancer center. *Neurosurgery*. 1999; 44: 74–79.

56. Subbarao K, Jacobson HG. Primary malignant neoplasms. *Sem Roentgenol*. 1979; 14: 44–57.

57. Pilepich MV, Vietti TJ, Nesbit ME, et al. Ewing's sarcoma of the vertebral column. *Int J Radiat Oncol Biol Phys*. 1981; 7: 27–31.

58. Sharfuddin MJA, Haddad FS, Hitchon PW, et al. Treatment options in primary Ewing's sarcoma of the spine: Report of seven cases and review of the literature. *Neurosurgery*. 1992; 30: 610–619.

59. Dydyk AM, Forro SD, Hanna A. Sacroiliac joint injury. StatPearls. https://www.ncbi.nlm.nih.gov/books/NBK557881/

60. Coccolini F, Stahel PF, Montori G, et al. Pelvic trauma: WSES classification and guidelines. *World J Emerg Surg*. 2017; 12: 5.

61. Day AC, Kinmont C, Bircher MD, Kumar S. Crescent fracture dislocation of the sacroiliac joint: A functional classification. *J Bone Joint Surg [Br]*. 2007; 89: 651–658.

62. Albert HB, Godskesen M, Westergaard JG. Incidence of four syndromes of pregnancy-related pelvic joint pain. *Spine*. 2002; 27 (24): 2831–2834.

63. Smith MW, Marcus PS, Wurtz LD. Orthopedic issues in pregnancy. *Obstet Gynecol Surv*. 2008; 63(2): 103–111.

3

Diagnostic evaluation of sacroiliac disease

Nicholas C. Canzanello and Jonathan M. Hagedorn

Introduction

Patients suffering from sacroiliac joint (SIJ) dysfunction may have symptoms that resemble those found in lumbar spine pathology. Because of this, proper diagnosis of SIJ pathology requires a thoughtful and thorough approach, including history, physical exam, imaging, and laboratory evidence. This chapter reviews the evidence supporting the diagnosis of different SIJ conditions.

Symptoms

Inciting factors

One study on patients with low back or buttock pain relieved after intraarticular SIJ injection found that 44% had a preceding traumatic event (such as a fall or motor vehicle accident), 21% had a cumulative injury (exercise related or altered gait), and 35% had an insidious onset of pain.[1]

Location

Patients typically describe buttock or posterior thigh pain. In one study, researchers injected the SIJ of 11 asymptomatic volunteers and documented hypesthesia and pain referral diagrams.[2] All volunteers developed pain within 10 cm inferior and 3 cm lateral to the posterior superior iliac spine (PSIS), as evident in Figure 3.1. Some volunteers also developed pain laterally to the superior greater trochanter and inferiorly into the lateral thigh.[2]

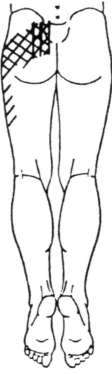

FIGURE 3.1. Composite referral map demonstrating overlap of sensory changes after SIJ injections in volunteers. *Source:* Reprinted with permission: Fortin JD, Aprill CN, Ponthieux B, Pier J. Sacroiliac joint: Pain referral maps upon applying a new injection/arthrography technique. Spine. 1994;19(13):1475–1482.

Inflammatory etiologies

In younger patients with low back and/or buttock pain, a detailed history must be obtained in an effort to screen for features suggestive of spondyloarthropathy, which is a group of inflammatory spine diseases including ankylosing spondylitis, psoriatic arthritis, reactive arthritis, arthritis associated with inflammatory bowel disease, and undifferentiated spondyloarthritis.[3] A 2006 study of 213 patients under the age of 50 with chronic back pain proposed a combination of parameters to screen for ankylosing spondylitis:

- Morning stiffness of more than 30 minutes duration
- Improvement in back pain with exercise but not with rest
- Awakening because of back pain during the second half of the night only
- Alternating buttock pain.[4]

When two of the four parameters were present, the sensitivity was 70.3%, with a specificity of 81.2%.[4] In the same study, it was noted that back pain onset under the age of 35 was more frequent in patients with ankylosing spondylitis than patients with mechanical back pain.[4]

Physical exam

Palpation of SIJ

The SIJ starts directly medial to the PSIS and extends inferiorly several centimeters. In a 1997 study published in *Spine*, tenderness over the sacral sulcus, just medial of the PSIS, was the most sensitive test for diagnosis of SIJ pain established by SIJ injection with an anesthetic.[5]

Reliability of physical exam maneuvers

Historically, there have been six fundamental physical exam maneuvers for the provocation of SIJ pain:

- FABER/Patrick test
- Gaenslen test
- Distraction
- Thigh thrust
- Compression
- Sacral thrust

A 2005 study by Laslett et al. found that using a threshold of three positive out of five commonly used SIJ pain provocation tests (distraction, compression, thigh thrust, sacral thrust, Gaenslen) had a sensitivity of 93.8% and a specificity of 78.1%.[6] This was reinforced when van der Wurff et al. published results that using a threshold of three positive out of five commonly used SIJ pain provocation tests (distraction, compression, thigh thrust, FABER, Gaenslen) had a sensitivity of 85% (95% confidence interval [CI]: 72–99%) and a specificity of 79% (95% CI: 65–93%).[7] However, a more recent study by Schneider et al. in 2020 found that no single physical exam maneuver, nor any combination of maneuvers, was associated with response to SIJ injection with anesthetic.[8] Two additional studies (Maigne et al. and Dreyfuss et al.) found no statistically significant association between response to SIJ anesthetic injection and any physical exam maneuvers.[9,10] Table 3.1 shows the sensitivity and specificity of common physical exam maneuvers for the provocation of SIJ pain.

Specific exam maneuvers

Distraction test

Conventionally, this test is performed with the patient in a supine position on the exam table. Using both hands to simultaneously palpate the bilateral anterior superior iliac spine, the clinician then applies a posteriorly directed force toward the table (Figure 3.2). This causes SIJ distraction. Pain with distraction is indicative of SIJ dysfunction.

Gaenslen test

The patient is supine with the ipsilateral leg hanging off the examination table and the contralateral knee and hip flexed. As demonstrated in Figure 3.3, one of the examiner's hands

TABLE 3.1 Sensitivity and specificity of seven physical exam maneuvers for the provocation of SIJ pain in separate studies

Study		FABER	Distraction	Thigh thrust	Gaenslen	Sacral thrust	Compression	Distraction PSIS
Laslett et al., 2005[6]	Sensitivity		0.60	0.88	0.53 (R SIJ) 0.50 (L SIJ)	0.63	0.69	
	Specificity		0.81	0.69	0.71 (R SIJ) 0.77 (L SIJ)	0.75	0.69	
Schneider et al., 2020[8]	Sensitivity	0.77	0.35	0.29	0.29	0.77	0.35	
	Specificity	0.28	0.83	0.72	0.44	0.28	0.78	
Werner et al., 2013[10]	Sensitivity							1.0
	Specificity							0.89

is used to apply a posterosuperior force to the contralateral leg while applying a downward, posterior force to the patient's ipsilateral, free-hanging leg. This maneuver is not advised in a patient with a hip replacement. If the patient's pain is reproduced in the ipsilateral SIJ, the test is considered positive.

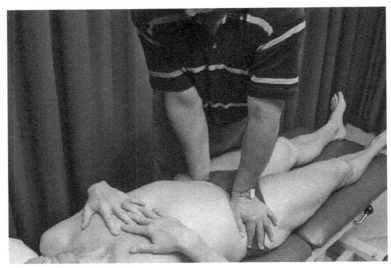

FIGURE 3.2. Distraction test. The posteriorly directed force applied by the examiner to the bilateral ASIS is stressing both SIJ. *Source:* Reprinted with permission: Laslett M. Evidence-based diagnosis and treatment of the painful sacroiliac joint. J Man Manip Ther. 2008;16(3):142–152.

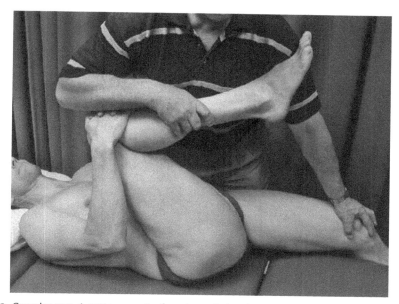

FIGURE 3.3. Gaenslen test. A posterosuperior force is applied to the contralateral leg while applying a downward, posterior force to the patient's ipsilateral, free-hanging leg to stress the ipsilateral SIJ. *Source:* Reprinted with permission: Laslett M. Evidence-based diagnosis and treatment of the painful sacroiliac joint. J Man Manip Ther. 2008;16(3):142–152.

FABER test

Also known as the Patrick test, this maneuver is performed with the patient supine. With the examiner's hand on the contralateral anterior superior iliac spine to stabilize the pelvis, the examiner **fl**exes, **ab**ducts, and **e**xternally **r**otates (hence the FABER acronym) the ipsilateral hip (Figure 3.4). Reported groin pain during this maneuver suggests intraarticular hip pathology, whereas pain over the SIJ or buttock suggests SIJ pathology. Other reported areas of pain are less specific.

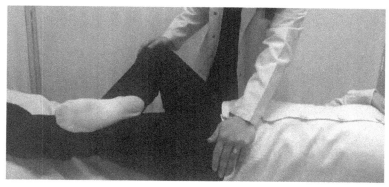

FIGURE 3.4. FABER/Patrick test. With the examiner's hand on the contralateral ASIS to stabilize the pelvis, the examiner flexes, abducts, and externally rotates the ipsilateral hip, stressing the ipsilateral SIJ. *Source:* Reprinted with permission: Telli H, Telli S, Topal M. The validity and reliability of provocation tests in the diagnosis of sacroiliac joint dysfunction. Pain Physician. 2018;21(4):E367–E376.

Thigh thrust test

With the patient supine, the examiner places one hand between the table and the patient's sacrum for stabilization. Using the other hand, the examiner brings the patient's hip into 90 degrees of flexion and an axial load (vertically oriented toward the table) is applied, stressing the ipsilateral SIJ (Figure 3.5).[11,12] This position is similar to the labral scour test of the hip, which also stresses the hip joint.

Compression test

With the patient in a lateral recumbent position with hips and knees bent, the examiner places downward force on the iliac crest directed toward the floor (Figure 3.6). The force is applied transversely across the pelvis, compressing the bilateral SIJs.[12] Reproducible pain is indicative of SIJ dysfunction.

Sacral thrust test

With the patient in a prone position, the examiner's thenar eminence is placed at the apex of the curve of the sacrum.[12] The examiner's other hand is applied over the hand on the sacrum for support. Vertically oriented pressure toward the table is applied to the sacrum in order to stress the bilateral SIJs (Figure 3.7). Reproducible pain is indicative of SIJ dysfunction.

Drop test

Unlike the other tests described in this chapter, the drop test is an active provocation test. While standing upright with hands on a wall for stabilization and knees in full extension,

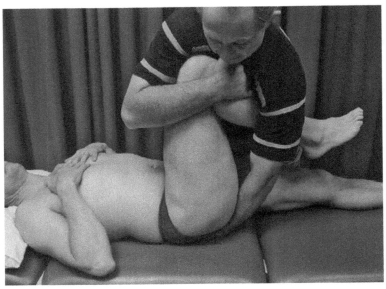

FIGURE 3.5. Thigh thrust test. The patient's hip is brought into 90 degrees of flexion and a downward force is applied, stressing the ipsilateral SIJ.[11,12] *Source:* Reprinted with permission: Laslett M. Evidence-based diagnosis and treatment of the painful sacroiliac joint. J Man Manip Ther. 2008;16(3):142–152.

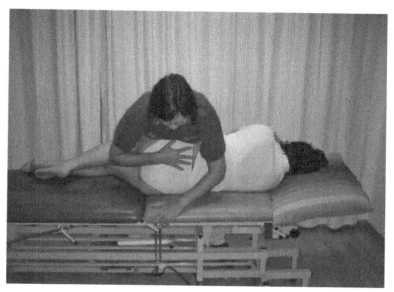

FIGURE 3.6. Compression test. With the patient in a lateral recumbent position with hips and knees bent, the examiner places downward force on the iliac crest directed toward the floor, stressing the bilateral SIJs.[12] *Source:* Reprinted with permission: Robinson HS, Brox JI, Robinson R, et al. The reliability of selected motion and pain provocation tests for the sacroiliac joint. Man Ther. 2007;12(1):72–79.

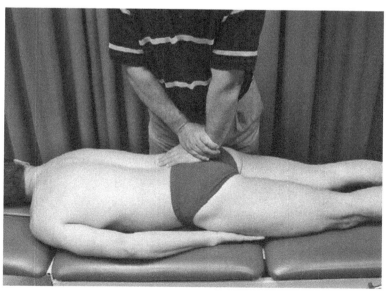

FIGURE 3.7. Sacral thrust test. Vertically oriented pressure toward the table is applied to the sacrum in order to stress the bilateral SIJs. *Source:* Reprinted with permission: Laslett M. Evidence-based diagnosis and treatment of the painful sacroiliac joint. J Man Manip Ther. 2008;16(3):142–152.

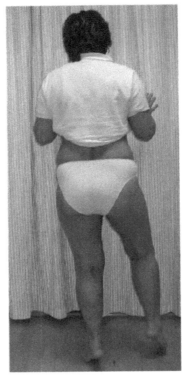

FIGURE 3.8. Drop test. A superior shear force to the ipsilateral SIJ is created by the patient suddenly dropping their raised heel to the floor while stabilized against a wall and keeping their knee extended and weight shifted to the ipsilateral side. *Source:* Reprinted with permission: Robinson HS, Brox JI, Robinson R, et al. The reliability of selected motion and pain provocation tests for the sacroiliac joint. Man Ther. 2007;12(1):72–79.

the patient raises one heel off the floor and shifts their weight to the same side (Figure 3.8). Then, by suddenly dropping the heel to the floor with continued knee extension, a superior shear force is created at the calcaneus into the ipsilateral SIJ.[12,13]

Distraction PSIS test

This test was first described in an article from Zurich, Switzerland, and is less commonly performed. With the patient either in a standing or a prone position, a punctual force is applied on the PSIS in a medial to lateral direction.[10] If the patient reports exacerbation of pain or development of new pain, the test is considered positive. In the single study out of Switzerland involving 46 patients, the reported sensitivity for SIJ pathology was 100% with a specificity of 89%.[10]

Schober test

In patients with an earlier onset of buttock pain or other historical features suggestive of inflammatory etiology, a Schober test can be performed. This examination maneuver is performed by marking the spine at the level of the iliac crest. Another mark is made 10 cm superior or cephalad from the first mark.[3] The patient is then asked to bend forward at the waist with straight knees. While the patient holds this position, the examiner measures the distance between the two marks. A change in distance between the two marks of greater than 5 cm is considered normal spinal mobility.[3]

Diagnostic injections

Response to intraarticular SIJ block has been the accepted standard for the diagnosis of SIJ dysfunction for many years. However, there are known to be both intraarticular and extraarticular structures of the SIJ, all of which are potential pain generators.[14] In 1994, the International Association for the Study of Pain listed pain relief with local anesthetic injection into the symptomatic joint as a criterion for the diagnosis of SIJ pain, along with pain present in the region of the SIJ and reproduction of pain upon stressing the SIJ during physical exam maneuvers.[15,16]

Imaging

Radiographs

Radiographs are the most cost-effective imaging technique for evaluating suspected SIJ pain; however, the sensitivity is poor for detecting early arthritic changes when compared to computed tomography (CT) or magnetic resonance imaging (MRI) modalities.[17] The standard radiograph for SIJ evaluation is an anteroposterior (AP) pelvis radiograph, although other dedicated SIJ views have been proposed.[17,18] One of these alternative views is the Ferguson view, which is a modified AP view with 20 to 30 degrees of cephalad angulation.[17] However, in a 2017 study by Omar et al.,[18] the Ferguson view did not show superiority for diagnosis of sacroiliitis when compared to the standard AP pelvis view.

Early findings of osteoarthritis, including joint space narrowing, subchondral sclerosis, and osteophytes, can be identified with radiography.[17] Radiography can also be used as a screening measure for the diagnosis of spondyloarthropathy. Findings suggestive of sacroiliitis can include asymmetric blurring of cortical margins, erosions, sclerosis, and bony ankyloses.[3] Examples of these findings on radiography can be seen in Figure 3.9.

Ultrasound

Multiple descriptions of ultrasound-guided SIJ injection techniques exist. A 2013 article from Italy used ultrasound to show that SIJ width and sacrotuberous ligament thickness were higher in patients with early spondyloarthritis compared to matched controls.[19]

CT

In a 2017 study by Backlund et al., 123 patients with symptomatic SIJ degeneration and 123 asymptomatic controls underwent CT imaging. There was no significant correlation between degenerative CT changes of the SIJ and symptoms.[20] Degenerative changes of the SIJ can be identified by CT imaging. These changes include joint space narrowing, osteophytes, subchondral sclerosis, and subchondral cysts.[20] CT images of SIJ space narrowing and osteophyte development are seen in Figures 3.10, 3.11 and 3.12A. Elementary structural lesions

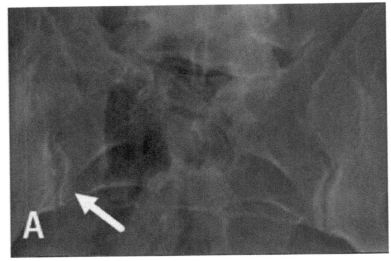

FIGURE 3.9. Radiograph showing grade 2 sacroiliitis on the right SIJ (*white arrow*) and grade 1 sacroiliitis on the left SIJ with isolated sclerosis.[21] *Source:* Reprinted with permission: Melchior J, Azraq Y, Chary-Valckenaere I, et al. Radiography, abdominal CT and MRI compared with sacroiliac joint CT in diagnosis of structural sacroiliitis. Eur J Radiol. 2017;95:169–176.

indicative of sacroiliitis, such as sclerosis, erosions, or change in joint space, can be detected by a dedicated SIJ CT or by abdominal CT imaging.[21]

MRI

MRI findings of sacroiliitis include bone marrow edema adjacent to the SIJ, gadolinium enhancement, sclerosis, and erosions.[3] As expected, the duration of back pain was significantly higher in those with radiographic findings definitive of sacroiliitis compared to those without.[4] MRI images showing progressive SIJ osteoarthritis are found in Figure 3.12B.

(A) (B) (C)

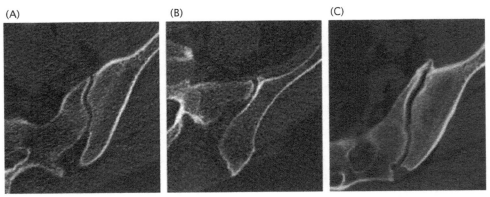

FIGURE 3.10. Axial CT images showing a left SIJ with no osteophytes (a), small osteophytes (b), and larger osteophytes (c). *Source:* Reprinted with permission: Backlund J, Clewett Dahl E, Skorpil M. Is CT indicated in diagnosing sacroiliac joint degeneration? Clin Radiol. 2017;72(8):693.e9–693.e13.

(A) (B) (C)

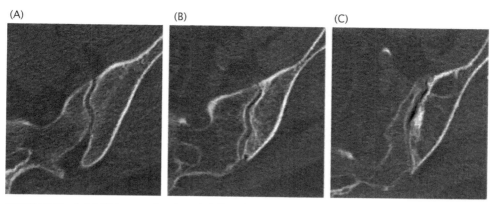

FIGURE 3.11. Axial CT images showing a left SIJ with no joint narrowing (a), focal joint narrowing (b), and more generalized joint narrowing (c). *Source:* Reprinted with permission: Backlund J, Clewett Dahl E, Skorpil M. Is CT indicated in diagnosing sacroiliac joint degeneration? Clin Radiol. 2017;72(8):693.e9–693.e13.

Laboratory evidence

When the clinician is concerned about an inflammatory etiology of SIJ pain, inflammatory markers (C-reactive protein and erythrocyte sedimentation rate) may be obtained, but elevation is nonspecific. Human leukocyte antigen B27 (HLA-B27) has been regarded as the most useful laboratory study for the diagnosis of ankylosing spondylitis.[3] In a study of 649 patients with chronic back pain with onset before 45 years of age, HLA-B27 was positive in 65.9% of patients who were ultimately diagnosed with an axial spondyloarthropathy and 27% of patients without spondyloathropathy.[4] In a separate study on patients with chronic

(A)

(B)

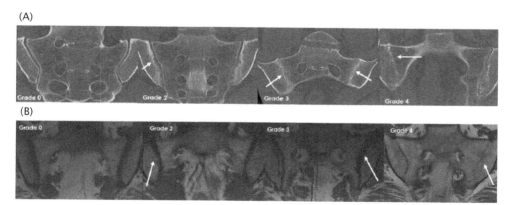

FIGURE 3.12. Radiographic evidence of elementary structural lesions of the SIJs on CT (**A**) and MRI (**B**) with scoring using the modified New York criteria.[21] (**A**) Grade 0 is represented by normal SIJs. Grade 2 shows sclerosis and erosions (*arrow*) of both SIJs. Grade 3 shows right sacroiliac joint space narrowing (*arrow*) and left SIJ partial ankylosis (*arrow*). Grade 4 shows total synostosis of the right SIJ.[21] (**B**) Grade 0 is represented by normal SIJs. Grade 2 shows iliac-sided erosions (*arrow*) of the right SIJ. Grade 3 shows erosions and widening (*arrow*) of the left SIJ. Grade 4 demonstrates total synostosis of the left SIJ. *Source:* Reprinted with permission: Melchior J, Azraq Y, Chary-Valckenaere I, et al. Radiography, abdominal CT and MRI compared with sacroiliac joint CT in diagnosis of structural sacroiliitis. Eur J Radiol. 2017;95:169–176.

back pain with onset before 45 years of age, HLA-B27 positivity had an odds ratio of 2.8 with axial spondyloarthropathy as the outcome.

Conclusion

Appropriately diagnosing SIJ dysfunction can be difficult, but it is imperative for proper treatment allocation and patient outcomes. The diagnosis involves a combination of thorough history, specific physical exam maneuvers, appropriate imaging, and bloodwork, if indicated. Often, a diagnostic intraarticular injection is necessary to confirm the diagnosis given the lack of sensitivity and specificity of physical exam maneuvers.

References

1. Chou LH, Slipman CW, Bhagia SM, et al. Inciting events initiating injection-proven sacroiliac joint syndrome. Pain Med. 2004;5(1):26–32.
2. Fortin JD, Aprill CN, Ponthieux B, Pier J. Sacroiliac joint: Pain referral maps upon applying a new injection/arthrography technique. Spine. 1994;19(13):1475–1482.
3. Harper BE, Reveille JD. Spondyloarthritis: Clinical suspicion, diagnosis, and sports. Curr Sports Med Rep. 2009;8(1):29–34. doi:10.1249/JSR.0b013e3181967ac6
4. Rudwaleit M, Metter A, Listing J, et al. Inflammatory back pain in ankylosing spondylitis: A reassessment of the clinical history for application as classification and diagnostic criteria. Arthritis Rheum. 2006;54(2):569–578. doi:10.1002/art.21619
5. Dreyfuss P, Michaelsen M, Pauza K, et al. The value of medical history and physical examination in diagnosing sacroiliac joint pain. Spine. 1996;21(22):2594–2602. doi:10.1097/00007632-199611150-00009
6. Laslett M, Aprill CN, McDonald B, Young SB. Diagnosis of sacroiliac joint pain: Validity of individual provocation tests and composites of tests. Man Ther. 2005;10(3):207–218. doi:10.1016/j.math.2005.01.003
7. van der Wurff P, Buijs EJ, Groen GJ. A multitest regimen of pain provocation tests as an aid to reduce unnecessary minimally invasive sacroiliac joint procedures. Arch Phys Med Rehabil. 2006;87(1):10–14. doi:10.1016/j.apmr.2005.09.023
8. Schneider BJ, Ehsanian R, Rosati R, et al. Validity of physical exam maneuvers in the diagnosis of sacroiliac joint pathology. Pain Med. 2020;21(2)255–260. doi:10.1093/pm/pnz183
9. Maigne JY, Aivaliklis A, Pfefer F. Results of sacroiliac joint double block and value of sacroiliac pain provocation tests in 54 patients with low back pain. Spine. 1996;21(16):1889–1892. doi:10.1097/00007632-199608150-00012
10. Werner C, Hoch A, Gautier L, et al. Distraction test of the posterior superior iliac spine (PSIS) in the diagnosis of sacroiliac joint arthropathy. BMC Surg. 2013;13:52.
11. Telli H, Telli S, Topal M. The validity and reliability of provocation tests in the diagnosis of sacroiliac joint dysfunction. Pain Physician. 2018;21(4):E367–E376.
12. Laslett M. Evidence-based diagnosis and treatment of the painful sacroiliac joint. J Man Manip Ther. 2008;16(3):142–152. doi:10.1179/jmt.2008.16.3.142
13. Robinson HS, Brox JI, Robinson R, et al. The reliability of selected motion and pain provocation tests for the sacroiliac joint. Man Ther. 2007;12(1):72–79.
14. Schneider BJ, Huynh L, Levin J, et al. Does immediate pain relief after an injection into the sacroiliac joint with anesthetic and corticosteroid predict subsequent pain relief? Pain Med. 2018;19(2):244–251. doi:10.1093/pm/pnx104

15. Merskey H, Bogduk N, International Association for the Study of Pain (Eds.). *Classification of chronic pain: Descriptions of chronic pain syndromes and definitions of pain terms* (2nd ed., p. 222). IASP Press, 1994.

16. Schneider BJ, Rosati R, Zheng P, McCormick ZL. Challenges in diagnosing sacroiliac joint pain: A narrative review. PM R. 2019;11(Suppl. 1):S40–S45. doi:10.1002/pmrj.12175

17. Tuite MJ. Sacroiliac joint imaging. Semin Musculoskelet Radiol. 2008;12(1):72–82. doi:10.1055/s-2008-1067939

18. Omar A, Sari I, Bedaiwi M, et al. Analysis of dedicated sacroiliac views to improve reliability of conventional pelvic radiographs. Rheumatology. 2017;56(10):1740–1745. https://doi.org/10.1093/rheumatology/kex240

19. Bandinelli F, Melchiorre D, Scazzariello F, et al. Clinical and radiological evaluation of sacroiliac joints compared with ultrasound examination in early spondyloarthritis. Rheumatology. 2013;52(7):1293–1297. doi:10.1093/rheumatology/ket105

20. Backlund J, Clewett Dahl E, Skorpil M. Is CT indicated in diagnosing sacroiliac joint degeneration? Clin Radiol. 2017;72(8):693.e9–693.e13. doi:10.1016/j.crad.2017.03.006

21. Melchior J, Azraq Y, Chary-Valckenaere I, et al. Radiography, abdominal CT and MRI compared with sacroiliac joint CT in diagnosis of structural sacroiliitis. Eur J Radiol. 2017;95:169–176. doi:10.1016/j.ejrad.2017.08.004

4

Disability associated with sacroiliac joint diseases

Lisa R. Kroopf, Kemly Philip,
Michelle N. Dang, and Samara Shipon

Introduction

Disability refers to the loss of function derived from an impairment, or the alteration of a physical structure, that limits one's performance of activities of daily living (ADLs) related to household, work, or community engagement.[1] Globally, lower back pain (LBP) affects more than 1.7 billion people worldwide and ranks among the top three causes of years lived with disability, globally, alongside headache and depressive disorders.[2,1] In the United States alone, at least 66 million individuals reported LBP, with a prevalence of 28 out of 100 persons in 2012.[1] Eighty-four percent of adults will experience LBP at some point in their lifetime, with up to 12% becoming disabled or incapable of substantial gainful employment.[3] Disabling LBP has a higher prevalence among individuals of low socioeconomic status. Sacroiliac joint (SIJ) pain is considered the primary source of pain in 14% to 22% of patients with axial LBP. It is reported in as many as 32% to 42% of patients with LBP with a history of lumbar fusion, as well as 49% among pregnant patients.[4,5] Point prevalence of SIJ pain is 15% to 30% with an annual prevalence of 20% to 60% and a lifetime prevalence of 60% to 70%.[6] The true epidemiology and impact of SIJ pain remain undefined in the literature. Thus, for the purpose of this chapter, specific data regarding disability from LBP as a whole have been extrapolated, in certain instances.

Risk factors for development of SIJ pain and dysfunction include factors that alter structural anatomy, including obesity, or increased mechanical forces on the SIJ complex due to mechanical or inflammatory causes, such as pregnancy or post-lumbar fusion (Box 4.1). Lumbar fusion surgery has been identified as a prominent risk factor for development of new-onset SIJ pain. In a study by Lee et al., of 317 patients who had undergone lumbar fusion surgery, 38 developed new-onset SIJ pain, with an overall incidence of 12.0%. There was a slightly higher predominance of new SIJ pain in patients with lumbosacral fusion versus lumbar fusion, with a range of onset from 6 to 48 months (mean 22 months) after

---

BOX 4.1. Predisposing factors for SIJ pain and dysfunction

- Obesity
- Pregnancy
- Trauma: loading and rotational forces
- Transitional anatomy or scoliosis
- Leg length discrepancies
- Inflammatory arthropathies
- Gait abnormalities
- Post lumbar spine fusion
- Female (3–4 times higher risk)
- Office-based occupation
- Prolonged sitting

---

lumbar fusion surgery. The annual incidence rate for developing new-onset SIJ pain following lumbar fusion was 3.5% within the first year.[7] Box 4.1 describes physical risk factors for development of SIJ pain and dysfunction.[7,8]

Some factors that appear to contribute to ongoing persistent LBP and disability include high pain intensity at onset, depressive mood, pain severity and functional impact, prior LBP episodes, psychological stress, or involvement of multiple sites of pain, which can lead to an exaggerated pain response.[9,3] Recent research suggests a role for centrally mediated pain-modulating mechanisms as well due to central sensitization driven by inflammation.[9]

Physical, physiologic, and psychosocial effects of SIJ pain

Physical effects

The largest axial joint in the body that connects the lumbar spine to the pelvis is the SIJ. The exact pattern of innervation of the SIJ is unclear; many experts have described innervation from the lateral branches of the L4–S3 dorsal rami.[4] There is significant variation among males and females in terms of anatomic structure and function of the pelvis, and these affect the biomechanics of the SIJ. The movement of the SIJ is more translational in males versus rotational in females. The sacral cartilage is thicker in females and thinner in males. The iliac bone cortical layer is thinner in females and thicker in males. The female pelvis is wider and shorter and the male pelvis is narrower and taller. The sciatic notch and the acetabula are wider in females and narrower in males. The pubic angle is larger (90–100 degrees) in females and smaller (50–80 degrees) in males. In females the interosseous sacroiliac ligament is larger than in males, whereas both the anterior and posterior sacroiliac ligaments are smaller.[10]

The ligaments that surround the SIJ as well as the pelvic floor muscles (levator ani and coccygeus muscles) provide stability and limit movement of the SIJ.[11] The movement of the sacrum in relation to the ilium is only 6 degrees. The posterior sacroiliac ligament provides the majority of movement of the sacrum, which is anterior and posterior tilt. Although numerous muscles surround the joint, they do not provide active activation of the joint. These muscles include the erector spinae, hamstrings, gluteals, psoas, quadratus lumborum, and piriformis.[10] The SIJ itself is a joint whose main function is to maintain stability, to transmit and decrease loads to the lower extremities, and to limit rotation of the body. Additionally, in women, the SIJ facilitates labor.[4]

Injury to the SIJ can be due to intraarticular causes or extraarticular causes. Intraarticular causes include arthritis or infection. Extraarticular causes include trauma such as fractures or ligamentous injury or myofascial pain. Of the two, extraarticular causes are more common.[4] SIJ pain can lead to both anatomic and physical effects such as SIJ ligament and joint tenderness, positional asymmetry due to pain or muscle tightness or weakness, dyspareunia, or changes in bladder function due to involvement of surrounding nerves.[11,12] Subsequent functional physical effects might include gait abnormalities, poor sitting tolerance, and the need for frequent position changes due to pain with transitional movements.[8] Other activity limitations include decreased ambulation, climbing, truncal twisting, or prolonged standing due to increased loading of the SIJ that may contribute to pain.[12]

Risk factors for developing SIJ pain include mechanical issues such as leg length discrepancies, gait disturbances, lumbar fusion, and scoliosis.[4] Pregnancy can lead to SIJ pain due to changes in posture, increased weight, trauma of labor, and ligament laxity from hormonal changes.[4] Furthermore, during pregnancy laxity in the dorsal ligament is the most common ligamentous source of pain due to its role in preventing posterior sacral tilt.[10]

Physiologic effects

To better understand the deleterious effects of a maladaptive response to chronic physiologic stress, it is important to review the underlying mechanisms involved in chronic pain processing and how these factors contribute to the persistence of pain and disability. The relationship between an overactive response to stress and chronic pain is well described by the sympathetic and neuroendocrine response to chronic stress. A stimulus that provokes fear, danger, or a perceived physical or psychological threat can elicit a short-term response that can serve an adaptive purpose to promote an individual's survival. In this phase, cortisol plays an essential role to prevent rampant inflammation that can result in widespread tissue and nerve damage. A balance between the sympathetic and parasympathetic response is key to long-term physical health, and it is believed that exacerbation of the acute physiologic stress response can, in fact, contribute to the development of chronic pain. For example, activation of the sympathetic mediators, including epinephrine and norepinephrine in the acute response, is typically followed by a delayed neuroendocrine response that includes cortisol dysfunction. Irrespective of a pain or non–pain-related stimulus, chronic

---

BOX 4.2. Psychosocial effects of SIJ pain

Behavioral manifestations:

- Maladaptive behaviors
- Fear-avoidance beliefs
- Pain catastrophizing
- Self-perceived disability
- Sensation of loss of control
- *Helplessness* → Mood disorders
- *Hopelessness* → Depression/anxiety

---

reactivation of this response leads to a maladaptive acute stress response that diminishes the subsequent cortisol response. Studies demonstrate that dysregulation of the neuroendocrine response can lead to stress-induced hypocortisolism, which in turn can result in multiorgan systemic effects. These effects include cognitive impairments on memory and attention, sleep disorders, and chronic pain disorders such as fibromyalgia, chronic fatigue syndrome, or chronic pelvic pain. Most importantly, decreased production of the anti-inflammatory cortisol can lead to increased systemic inflammation associated with diseases such as osteoporosis, rheumatoid arthritis, and chronic LBP.[13]

Box 4.2 describes the psychosocial effects of chronic SIJ pain that can contribute to the development of mood disorders, including depression.[14,13]

Psychosocial effects

The psychosocial effects related to chronic pain and LBP are substantial. The fear-avoidance model discusses two responses to an individual's experience of pain: fear avoidance and catastrophizing response. In the fear-avoidance response, an individual responding to a perceived trigger may try to avoid all social or recreational activities associated with that trigger. Patients who magnify their perception of pain in the catastrophizing response may also develop fear-avoidance behaviors to minimize their perceived triggers. If these behaviors are missed, then chronic disability can result (Figure 4.1).[14, 15,13] Fear-based memories of pain or stress can lead to anxiety and other mood disorders. Chronic pain that results in the sensation of loss of control and self-perceived disability may likewise result in feelings of helplessness and hopelessness that characterize depression (see Box 4.2).[15,12]

Appropriate treatment to minimize disability as a result of maladaptive behaviors typically involves cognitive-behavioral therapy with physical or occupational therapy services that employ confrontation to break the pain–fear–avoidance cycle. Importantly, creating an environment in which patients feel that their pain experience is validated, as though they have control over decisions related to their pain management, is pivotal in minimizing the development of fears associated with chronic SIJ pain. Psychosocial effects tie in closely with physiologic effects of pain as an exaggerated psychological response can increase cortisol

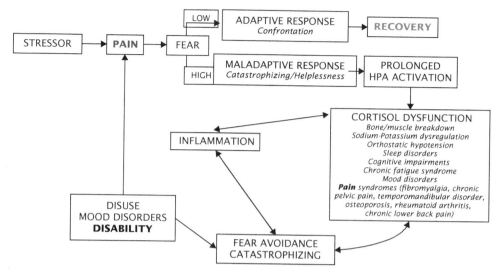

Adapted from the Fear Avoidance Model of Musculoskeletal Pain [15, 13].

FIGURE 4.1. Psychosocial consequences of the chronic physiologic stress response.

secretion, facilitating fear-based pain memories or stressors that ultimately can lead to an increased stress response when confronted with the same stimulus repeatedly.[13]

Burden of disability from LBP

LBP is a leading cause of activity limitation and missed work days globally, creating both substantial medical and economic impacts that vary depending on geographic health care costs, health care utilization, and perception of disability.[14,9,16] In developed countries, LBP is in fact one of the top three causes of disability, resulting in 83 million well-year of life lost.[17,2] An estimated 25.5 million individuals lost an average of 11.4 work days due to back and neck pain in 2012.[1] Furthermore, approximately 2.3% of physician visits are related to LBP in the United States, with health care costs estimated to exceed $100 billion; anually the average direct cost often exceeds $8,000 per individual per year. Lost productivity and increasing insurance premiums create a significant economic burden as well for patients with SIJ pain, along with society at large.[2,12]

In the United States, LBP is the most common cause for prescription opioid usage, which also poses a significant psychosocial and economic burden. Opioid dependence is an ongoing epidemic in the United States, with nearly 4 million cases in 2017 and 68% of drug-overdose deaths related to opioid use.[2,18] The Centers for Disease Control and Prevention estimate that up to $75.8 billion per year is lost due to opioid misuse.[19] Although there exists little evidence to support their effectiveness in this setting, opioids are often prescribed for acute LBP, with 13.7% of visits covered by private insurance resulting in a 7-day opioid prescription.[20] The large cohort study by Azad et al. noted that 27% of opioid-naive patients with newly diagnosed LBP received an opioid prescription.[20] According to evidence, acute or subacute LBP should be initially managed with modalities such as heat/ice, physical therapy, massage, acupuncture, or spinal manipulation as well as non-opioid medications such as nonsteroidal anti-inflammatories and/or muscle relaxants. Alternative treatments for chronic LBP include a multimodal approach that encompasses exercise and/or mind–body programs, motor control exercise, and biofeedback, with consideration of tramadol or duloxetine as second-line therapy. The American College of Physicians recommends opioids only for patients with chronic LBP who have failed to respond to conservative measures and the other drug classes just mentioned.[21] The poorly supported use of opioids in the management of acute and chronic LBP contributes to the substantial costs related to chronic back pain in terms of health care costs and lost productivity.[20] Pain perception overall is affected by the use of opioids, additionally leading to higher disability and lower quality of life.[16]

Patients with SIJ pain rated themselves to be in poor physical health in comparison to other disease states, reporting poor quality of life and greater decrements in health than other chronic diseases, including chronic obstructive pulmonary disease (COPD),[17,22] coronary artery disease, asthma, or mild heart failure.[17] When health utility values were compared among cohorts of patients with SIJ pain, studies found that the decrement in quality-of-life measures was more marked than other prominent spinal conditions (e.g., degenerative spondylolisthesis, spinal stenosis, and intervertebral disc herniation) in addition to other major diseases (e.g., liver cirrhosis and COPD). Health utility values were similar to orthopedic conditions such as hip and knee osteoarthritis. Oswestry Disability Index scores correlated inversely with quality-of-life measures among these cohorts. These findings suggest that SIJ pain leads to as much or higher levels of disability compared to other spinal conditions, and that careful physical examination and diagnostic methods should be used to ensure appropriate treatment is directed toward the underlying cause of pain and dysfunction.[22]

Disability evaluation

Functional assessment tools for disability due to LBP include the Oswestry Low Back Pain Disability Questionnaire, which evaluates how patients' pain may limit their ability for self-care, lifting, ambulation, sitting, standing, traveling, and social and sexual life.[23] The Western Ontario and McMaster Universities Arthritis Index (WOMAC) similarly assesses functional mobility and ADLs.[24] These tools can be used in conjunction with evaluation of joint mobility, motor function, range of motion, and sensation to help guide decisions on conservative versus interventional treatments for SIJ pain.[25]

The discussion of disability evaluations in this chapter is not meant to be exhaustive but rather an overview. The World Health Organization describes two more models, including the International Classification of Impairments, Disability, and Handicaps (ICIDH) alongside the International Classification of Functioning, Disability, and Health (ICF) model. Briefly, the prior 1999 ICIDH model recognizes four levels: (1) pathology, or the active disease process; (2) impairment at the organ level due to this pathology altering structure; (3) disability or activity limitation due to the impairment; and (4) handicap, or the societal restrictions due to the disability.[26] The more recent ICF, endorsed in 2001, has three parts: body function and structure, activity execution, and activity participation.[27] The Institute of Medicine model designates individuals as disabled if they meet criteria regarding medical impairment, functional limitations, work disability, non-work disability, and quality of life.[28]

Once an individual meets criteria for disability in these models, disability rating systems are critical to assess physical and functional losses at the point of medical maximal improvement (MMI) along with return-to-work restrictions. These ratings might then be used by workers' compensation or Social Security disability administrators to financially support covered workers who meet eligibility requirements, although there is no system by which full earnings are compensated.[29] Additional limitations to these rating systems include lack of validated ADL-based functional assessment tools in the context of varying medical impairments and poor metrics for vocational or non-vocational disability.[29,30]

Conclusion

SIJ pain has been described as a potential pain generator since as early as 1905.[7] SIJ pain and dysfunction is a global and public health problem that substantially contributes to increased health care and economic costs. Accurate diagnosis of SIJ pain and effective pain management using an appropriate multidisciplinary approach is critical in mitigating debilitating sequelae related to chronic pain leading to long-term disability. The remainder of this textbook addresses the anatomy, underlying causes, and treatments intended to prevent long-term disability from SIJ pain. Goals of inpatient and outpatient rehabilitation include reducing modifiable risk factors and using multimodal treatment plans to ultimately promote independence among patients with SIJ pain. Judicious and appropriate utilization of analgesics, bracing, injections, and advanced targeted pain therapies, in combination with identifying durable medical equipment and adaptive equipment needs, will ultimately help patients return to ADLs, mobility, and community reintegration.[25] Management of psychological and socioeconomic factors is also pivotal in mitigating potential chronic pain or a chronic stress response, as discussed earlier in the chapter. Ultimately, a greater response is required not only to improve access to health care and resources, but also to raise awareness of the disparities among burden of disease and public policies, research efforts and global initiatives aimed at reducing long-term disability, health care burden and economic costs.[9,16,1]

References

1. United States Bone and Joint Initiative. *The burden of musculoskeletal diseases in the United States* (3rd ed.). 2014. http://www.boneandjointburden.org.
2. Salomon JA, Vos T, Hogan DR, et al. Common values in assessing health outcomes from disease and injury: Disability weights measurement study for the Global Burden of Disease Study 2010. *Lancet.* 2012;*380*(9859):2129–2143.

3. Sanzarello I, Merlini L, Rosa MA, et al. Central sensitization in chronic low back pain: A narrative review. *J Back Musculoskelet Rehabil*. 2016;*29*(4):625–633. doi:10.3233/BMR-160685. PMID: 27062464.

4. Cohen SP, Chen Y, Neufeld NJ. Sacroiliac joint pain: A comprehensive review of epidemiology, diagnosis and treatment. *Expert Rev Neurother*. 2013;*13*(1):99–116. doi:10.1586/ern.12.148. PMID: 23253394.

5. Foley BS, Buschbacher RM. Sacroiliac joint pain: Anatomy, biomechanics, diagnosis, and treatment. *Am J Phys Med Rehabil*. 2006;*85*(12):997–1006. doi:10.1097/01.phm.0000247633.68694.c1. PMID: 17117004.

6. O'Shea FD, Boyle E, Salonen DC, et al. Inflammatory and degenerative sacroiliac joint disease in a primary back pain cohort. *Arthritis Care Res*. 2010;*62*(4):447–454. doi:10.1002/acr.20168. PMID: 20391497.

7. Lee YC, Lee R, Harman C. The incidence of new onset sacroiliac joint pain following lumbar fusion. *J Spine Surg*. 2019;*5*(3):310–314. doi:10.21037/jss.2019.09.05

8. Siahaan Y, Hartoyo V. Sacroiliac joint pain: A study of predisposing factors in an Indonesian hospital. *Open Pain J*. 2019;*12*:1–5. doi:10.2174/1876386301912010001

9. Hartvigsen J, Hancock MJ, Kongsted A, et al. What low back pain is and why we need to pay attention. *Lancet*. 2018;*391*(10137):2356–2367. doi: 10.1016/S0140-6736(18)30480-X. PMID: 29573870.

10. Kiapour A, Joukar A, Elgafy H, et al. Biomechanics of the sacroiliac joint: Anatomy, function, biomechanics, sexual dimorphism, and causes of pain. *Int J Spine Surg*. 2020;*14*(1):S3–S13.

11. Casaroli G, Bassani T, Brayda-Bruno M, et al. What do we know about biomechanics of the sacroiliac joint and sacroiliac joint fixation? A literature review. *Med Eng Phys*. 2020;*76*:1–12. doi:10.1016/j.medengphy.2019.10.009. PMID: 31866118.

12. Barros G, McGrath L, Gelfenbeyn M. Sacroiliac joint dysfunction in patients with low back pain. *Fed Pract*. 2019;*36*(8):370–375.

13. Hannibal KE, Bishop MD. Chronic stress, cortisol dysfunction, and pain: A psychoneuroendocrine rationale for stress management in pain rehabilitation. *Phys Ther*. 2014;*94*(12):1816–1825. doi:10.2522/ptj.20130597. PMID: 25035267; PMCID: PMC4263906.

14. La Touche R, Pérez-Fernández M, Barrera-Marchessi I, et al. Psychological and physical factors related to disability in chronic low back pain. *J Back Musculoskelet Rehabil*. 2019;*32*(4):603–611. doi:10.3233/BMR-181269. PMID: 30584119.

15. Leeuw M, Goossens ME, Linton SJ, et al. The fear-avoidance model of musculoskeletal pain: Current state of scientific evidence. *J Behav Med*. 2007;*30*(1):77–94.

16. Dengler J, Sturesson B, Kools D, et al. Risk factors for continued opioid use in conservative versus surgical management of low back pain originating from the sacroiliac joint. *Global Spine J*. 2018;*8*(5):453–459.

17. Cher D, Polly D, Berven S. Sacroiliac joint pain: Burden of disease. *Med Devices*. 2014;*7*:73–81. doi:10.2147/MDER.S59437

18. Wilson N, Kariisa M, Seth P, et al. Drug and opioid-involved overdose deaths—United States, 2017–2018. *MMWR Morb Mortal Wkly Rep*. 2020;*69*:290–297. http://dx.doi.org/10.15585/mmwr.mm6911a4

19. Florence CS, Zhou C, Luo F, Xu L. The economic burden of prescription opioid overdose, abuse, and dependence in the United States, 2013. *Med Care*. 2016;*54*(10):901–906. doi:10.1097/MLR.0000000000000625

20. Azad TD, Zhang Y, Stienen MN, et al. Patterns of opioid and benzodiazepine use in opioid-naïve patients with newly diagnosed low back and lower extremity pain. *J Gen Intern Med*. 2020;*35*(1):291–297. doi:10.1007/s11606-019-05549-8

21. Qaseem A, Wilt TJ, McLean RM, et al. Noninvasive treatments for acute, subacute, and chronic low back pain: A clinical practice guideline from the American College of Physicians. *Ann Intern Med*. 2017;*166*(7):514–530. doi:10.7326/M16-2367.PMID: 28192789.

22. Cher DJ, Reckling WC. Quality of life in preoperative patients with sacroiliac joint dysfunction is at least as depressed as in other lumbar spinal conditions. *Med Devices*. 2015;*8*:395–403. doi:10.2147/MDER.S92070

23. Fairbank JC, Pynsent PB. The Oswestry Disability Index. *Spine*. 2000;*25*(22):2940–2952.

24. Western Ontario and McMaster Universities Osteoarthritis Index. Shirley Ryan Ability Lab—Rehabilitation Measures Database. https://www.sralab.org/rehabilitation-measures/womac-osteoarthritis-index-reliability-validity-and-responsiveness-patients

25. Coats T, Dong X. SI joint pain. *Pain/Neuromuscular Medicine Rehabilitation.* Originally published: December 9, 2011; last updated: May 29, 2018. https://now.aapmr.org/si-joint-pain/

26. World Health Organization, Assessment, Classification and Epidemiology Unit. *International Classification of Functioning and Disability: ICIDH-2, Beta-2 draft, short version.* July 1999. https://apps.who.int/iris/handle/10665/65990

27. World Health Organization, Fifty-fourth World Health Assembly. International Classification of Functioning, Disability, and Health (ICF). May 22, 2001. https://www.who.int/classifications/icf/en/

28. Field MJ, Jetter AM (Eds.). *The future of disability in America.* Institute of Medicine (U.S.) Committee on Disability in America. National Academies Press, 2007.

29. Kareen A. Velez. Disability evaluation. *Essentials of Rehabilitation Practice and Science.* PM&R KnowledgeNOW. Originally published: October 22, 2013; last updated: December 1, 2020. https://now.aapmr.org/disability-evaluation/

30. Iezzoni LI, Freedman VA. Turning the disability tide: The importance of definitions. *JAMA.* 2008;299(3):332–334. doi:10.1001/jama.299.3.332. PMID: 18212318.

5

Types of anesthesia for different sacroiliac joint interventions

Behnum A. Habibi, Mark N. Malinowski, and Chong H. Kim

Introduction

Given the variety of interventional and surgical procedures performed for sacroiliac joint (SIJ) pain, there are many commonly used anesthetic techniques to be considered. After a brief discussion of the history of anesthesia in relation to SIJ procedures, this chapter will review common anesthetic options and their use in different procedures. For example, diagnostic SIJ injections do not necessitate anesthesia, while open SIJ fusions require general anesthesia. The chapter will discuss these and other techniques in order of increasing sedation. Local anesthesia will be discussed for intraarticular joint injections, blocks of the nerves innervating the SIJ, and radiofrequency ablations (RFAs) of these same nerves. Monitored anesthesia care (MAC) will be discussed for procedures such as minimally invasive SIJ fusions and the Simplicity RFA technique. The use of neuraxial anesthesia, via either spinal or epidural blocks, will be considered for lateral SIJ fusions. Finally, the use of general anesthesia for lateral and open fusions will be reviewed.

History of anesthesia for SIJ procedures

Local anesthetics date to the 1800s, when cocaine was used for surgical anesthesia. Cocaine is an alkaloid voltage-gated sodium ion channel blocker and was found originally in coca leaves before being synthesized by organic chemists in the late 1800s. By blocking the voltage-gated sodium ion channels in neural membranes, sodium ion conductance across the cell membrane is reduced. This results in stabilization of the membrane potential and inhibition of action potential generation and potentiation, thereby producing a reversible blockade of sensation and, at sufficient doses, motor activity. The adverse effects associated with cocaine prompted the development of novel sodium ion channel–blocking anesthetics. In 1905, procaine became available as a local anesthetic. However, its use in patients was associated with severe allergic reactions. In 1946, lidocaine became available and is still a popular local amide anesthetic.

The SIJ was first described by Bernhard Siegfried Albinus (1697–1770) and William Hunter (1718–1783).[1] While opinions differ regarding the nature of the joint and its classification, Von Luschka's 1864 description of it as a true diarthrodial joint is still popular. The joint was described as a source of low back pain by Goldwaith and Osgood in 1905.[2] Fortin et al. built on this concept by creating pain referral patterns elicited by contrast dye injections into the SIJ of asymptomatic volunteers.[3] The patterns were verified with subsequent local anesthetic injections into the joint. Anesthesia for SIJ injections has been used in a variety of ways since then. Most early procedures involved only local anesthesia. As the complexity of SIJ procedures has increased, more sedating forms of anesthesia have been used. Local anesthesia is used for blocks of the nerves supplying innervation to the SIJ. These blocks traditionally target the L5 dorsal ramus and lateral branches of the S1–3 nerve roots, though the posterior aspect of the SIJ is innervated by a plexus formed from the dorsal rami of L5–S4.[4] Innervation to the anterior aspect of the SIJ is not targeted in such blocks as its contribution to pain is not as well established and its innervation is more variable (usually L4–S2 nerve segments, though it may include L3 contributions, the sacral plexus, and, in a single anatomic study, the superior gluteal nerve). RFA of the nerves to the posterior SIJ has not been as well studied as nerve blocks, but retrospective, prospective, and randomized controlled trials of their efficacy have been reported since the 2000s. Typically local anesthesia is used for these ablations. When nerve blocks and ablations do not adequately control pain or are otherwise not therapeutic options, SIJ fusions can be performed, but these surgeries require more sedating anesthesia.

Historically, joint arthrodesis has been an open surgical procedure requiring general anesthesia. Like local anesthetics, general anesthesia has a history dating back to the 1800s. The first known use of diethyl ether was on March 30, 1842, by Crawford Long. It was a major breakthrough and marks the foundation of modern anesthesia and surgery.[5] Chloroform, another early general anesthetic, was famously used by Sir James Y. Simpson to provide analgesia to Queen Victoria in 1853 during the birth of Prince Leopold.[6] In relation to SIJ procedures, the risks associated with open surgeries have prompted the development of minimally invasive techniques that limit movement at the SIJ and reduce low back pain, limiting both the need for general anesthesia and postoperative morbidity. Multiple retrospective and prospective studies on the efficacy of minimally invasive fusions have been published since 2008.[7] Percutaneous fusions can be performed with either regional or general anesthesia. The remainder of this chapter will discuss these different anesthetic techniques in order of increasing sedation.

Anesthetic options for SIJ procedures
No anesthesia

The least sedating form of anesthesia is no anesthesia at all. This is the standard of care for diagnostic SIJ injections. The diagnostic SIJ injection involves the injection of anesthetic into the SIJ. The purpose of the injection is to narrow the differential in cases of low back or buttock pain. By instilling a small amount of local anesthetic in the joint, a positive response (i.e., a reduction in pain scores) can serve as a confirmatory diagnostic test for SIJ pain with high specificity. Lidocaine, typically 1% (though higher concentrations may be used), is most often used for diagnostic injections, given its rapid onset and short duration of action. Data from multiple studies gathered by the American Society of Anesthesiologists Task Force on Chronic Pain Management and the American Society of Regional Anesthesia and Pain Medicine demonstrate that the positive predictive value of the procedure is between 19% and 75% for pain of sacroiliac origin.[8] The sensitivity of this test would be negatively affected by any concomitant anesthesia. Furthermore, current techniques allow for the procedure to be comfortably performed without sedation or other anesthesia. For example, diagnostic SIJ injections can be performed using a 22- or 25-gauge spinal needle guided directly, with ultrasound or fluoroscopy,[9] to the posterior-inferior aspect of the joint.

Evidence directly supporting this technique can be extrapolated from the literature on other interventional pain procedures. For example, in 2019 Chen et al. published a prospective observational trial in *Pain Medicine* examining lumbar medial branch blocks performed with 25-gauge spinal needles.[10] The group investigated whether the procedure was more or less painful when performed with local anesthetic injected into the skin. Ninety-nine consecutive patients were included in the study (obese patients and those requiring larger needles were excluded). Patients rated the pain of each needle stick immediately following the multilevel blocks. Comparing 306 total needle sticks, the group found that the 25-gauge spinal needles placed with local anesthetic skin wheals were more painful on the whole than those placed without skin wheals ($p = .007$). Applying the findings of this study to SIJ procedures is limited by the different anatomic target as well as the substantial differences in the procedures themselves (number of needle sticks, crossing of joint capsules, contrast use, etc.). However, one may infer that other low back injections, such as diagnostic SIJ injections, performed with 25-gauge spinal needles are less painful when administered without local anesthesia.

In addition to patient comfort, a concern about using local anesthetics in diagnostic SIJ injections is their effect on sensitivity and specificity. Again, we can extrapolate from evidence on other lumbar spine procedures. Ackerman et al. compared different forms of anesthesia in lumbar facet joint injections in 2004.[11] Seventy-five males were recruited into their study, then assigned to one of five groups (Table 5.1). Patients in the groups receiving intramuscular injections superficial to the target joint (in this case the lumbar facet joint) had more pain relief than those receiving joint injections alone. The authors concluded that this may lead to false-positive results in diagnostic facet joint injections. Generalizing these findings to the SIJ is limited again by the variations in anatomy and differences in techniques. However, if one infers that intramuscular local anesthesia can provide pain relief for

TABLE 5.1 Comparison of groups in the Ackerman et al. study (2004) comparing different forms of local anesthesia prior to lumbar facet joint injections

Group I	Facet joint injection with continuous lidocaine administration from the skin to the facet joint as the needle was advanced
Group II	Facet joint injection with saline administration from the skin to the facet joint as the needle was advanced
Group III	Median nerve branch injection with a lidocaine advancing needle technique
Group IV	Median nerve branch injection with saline advancing needle technique
Group V	Injection of the paraspinous muscles with local anesthetic and steroid following noted areas of pain diagnosed with saline injection and radiopaque contrast

pathologic underlying joints, the use of intramuscular local anesthesia prior to a diagnostic SIJ injection may provide pain relief that masks the intended effects of the procedure. This is a particularly salient point given the importance of diagnostic blocks in predicting the success of radiofrequency procedures,[12] which will be discussed in additional detail later in this chapter. Thus, to preserve the sensitivity of the test, and given its well-tolerated nature, the diagnostic SIJ injection precludes the need for local anesthesia.

For patients requiring some form of pain treatment prior to any needle insertion, vapocoolants are reasonable alternatives to local anesthetics. The sprays have a rapid onset of action and are less likely to confound results of diagnostic SIJ testing. Data regarding vapocoolant use for SIJ procedures are not currently available, but a Cochrane review of vapocoolant use for intravenous cannulation was published in 2016.[13] Nine studies involving 1,070 patients were included in the review. The use of vapocoolants was shown to improve pain scores by 12.5 mm (0 mm = no pain, 100 mm = worst pain possible) when used immediately prior to needle insertion and did not affect the ease of performing the procedure or adverse events. The overall quality of the evidence was moderate. Therefore, it is likely that vapocoolant spray can be used prior to needle insertion not only for diagnostic SIJ procedures but also for any of the other SIJ procedures discussed in this chapter where patients may be awake for the beginning of the case.

Local anesthesia

Therapeutic SIJ intraarticular injections can be performed with different anesthetic agents. Bupivacaine and ropivacaine, which will be discussed at length in this section, are among the other most commonly used anesthetics for these intraarticular injections. Often, one of these anesthetics is combined with a steroid prior to injection into the joint. Given the joint's limited volume, 2 to 3 cc of anesthetic is used with 1 to 2 cc of steroid solution. Lidocaine, again typically 1%, is also useful as a rapid-onset local anesthetic subcutaneously prior to intraarticular injections. This is done by giving 2 to 5 cc directly under the skin. Subcutaneous lidocaine can be painful and may benefit from either local co-administration with sodium bicarbonate (which raises the pH and thereby reduces the burning sensation) or by warming the lidocaine solution to body temperature (being careful to avoid substantial heat, which can denature the anesthetic). Warming of local anesthetics was reviewed in a 2011 systematic review and meta-analysis of subcutaneous and intradermal anesthetic injections.[14] Eight hundred thirty-one patients were included in the meta-analysis of 19 randomized or pseudorandomized trials. On a 100-mm visual analog scale, the mean difference of 11 mm favored warming injections of local anesthetics over the control group. A meta-analysis of buffered versus non-buffered lidocaine for dental injections was published in 2018, favoring buffered solutions by 5 mm on the 100-mm visual analog scale.[15]

In addition to SIJ intraarticular injections, nerve blocks that target the L5 dorsal ramus and S1–3 lateral branches are an alternative option for the treatment of SIJ pain. Lidocaine is typically used subcutaneously in these procedures prior to insertion of needles to the target sites on or near the nerves. After confirmation of the needle-tip location, longer-acting local anesthetics are placed directly over the nerves, typically bupivacaine or ropivacaine. Volumes may vary by practitioner given the anatomic variability of the lateral branches of the S1–3 nerve roots. Lidocaine is not the best choice for the nerve block itself given its lower affinity for protein binding and thus shorter duration of action (discussed in more detail later in this chapter).

RFA of the lateral branches of the sacral nerve roots can serve as a longer-acting treatment for patients who have relief with nerve blocks. Local anesthesia for RFA typically consists of 1% lidocaine subcutaneously, again about 3 to 5 cc under the skin of the entry site. After needle placement is confirmed and prior to nerve ablation, local anesthesia is applied over these nerves to prevent pain during and after the procedure. Typically, bupivacaine or ropivacaine is used, given their longer duration of action. Lidocaine may be used in addition to the longer-acting anesthetic at this step to provide more rapid anesthesia over the nerves, shortening the overall procedure time. After the ablation, additional local anesthesia is often applied, with or without steroids. The proposed purpose of the steroid is to minimize the risk of post-ablation neuritis as well as to provide local anesthesia.

The remainder of this section will discuss the anesthetics commonly used for these and other SIJ procedures (Table 5.2.

The three most important factors that dictate the effects of local anesthetics are lipid binding, protein binding, and pKa:

- Lipid binding can affect potency as it correlates with the amount of drug that can penetrate cell membranes and bind sodium ion channels. For example, bupivacaine is more lipophilic than lidocaine and is about 10 times more potent.
- Protein binding affects the duration of drug availability in the plasma and thus the duration of action.
- pKa determines the amount of nonionic drug that is free to cross membranes and thus affects the onset timing. Lidocaine is a weak base, and as a result about 25% of in vivo lidocaine is available nonionized and free to cross membranes. Thus, lidocaine has a rapid onset time compared to other local anesthetics with a higher pKa.

TABLE 5.2 Comparison of local anesthetics commonly used for SIJ procedures

Anesthetic	Lidocaine	Bupivacaine	Ropivacaine
Chemical structure			
Onset	45–90 seconds as single systemic dose (route and dose dependent)	Fast (route and dose dependent)	3–5 minutes (route dependent)
Duration of action	10–20 minutes as single systemic dose (route and dose dependent)	1.5–8 hours (route and dose dependent)	3–15 hours (route and dose dependent)
Metabolism	Hepatic via CYP	Hepatic via CYP	Hepatic via CYP
Clearance	Adults: 640 ± 1.8 mL/min Children/infants: N/A	Adults: N/A Children: 10 ± 0.7 mL/kg/ minute Infants: 7.1 ± 3.2 mL/kg/ minute	387 ± 107 mL/min
Half-life	Biphasic: initial 7–30 minutes; secondary 1.5–2 hours (3.2 hours in infants)	2.7 hours (8.1 hours in neonates)	4.2 hours
Protein binding	60–80%	95%	94%
pKa	7.9	8.1	8.1

Lidocaine is a synthesized aminoethylamide, commonly referred to as an amide anesthetic.[16] It is a white or slightly yellow powder often manufactured as a hydrochloride salt in a 5% dextrose solution. The duration of action of lidocaine varies by the route of administration. Intravenously, lidocaine anesthetic effects last 10 to 20 minutes, while intramuscular injection provides 60 to 90 minutes of anesthesia. Many factors affect the local concentration of lidocaine in vivo and subsequently its duration of action. It is readily absorbed across mucous membranes, the upper and lower airways, and damaged skin but is only poorly absorbed across intact skin. Despite its permeability across mucous membranes, the bioavailability is only about 35%, given the high degree of first-pass metabolism. Among the injected routes, aside from intravenous injection, intercostal nerve blocks produce the highest blood concentrations, followed by injection into the lumbar epidural space, the brachial plexus, then subcutaneous tissue.

The local concentration of available amide anesthetics is affected by the local pH and degree of vasoconstriction, both of which can be manipulated by co-administration with epinephrine. By lowering the pH and contracting small blood vessels, epinephrine increases the local effect of lidocaine. The two are often co-administered in a solution as 2%

lidocaine with a 1:100,000 (0.01 mg/mL) or 1:50,000 (0.02 mg/mL) solution of epinephrine. The combination also provides the added benefit of reduced plasma lidocaine levels and thus reduced risk of systemic toxicity.

Lidocaine is metabolized by the liver and excreted by the kidney. Some metabolites act similarly to lidocaine but with less potency. The elimination half-life is approximately 1.5 to 2 hours, though it may be prolonged (up to twofold) in patients with liver failure. The maximum dose, with regard to systemic toxicity, of lidocaine is 4.5 mg/kg (without epinephrine), not to exceed 300 mg. Using 1% lidocaine as an example (equivalent to 10 mg/mL), 300 mg of lidocaine would equate to 30 mL.

Bupivacaine is also an amide anesthetic, structurally similar to lidocaine.[17] It is available as a hydrochloride salt in 0.25%, 0.5%, and 0.75% solutions in either 5% or 8% dextrose. The 0.75% solution is no longer recommended for obstetric patients due to serious adverse cardiovascular events that have occurred and may have been due to intravascular injection. Bupivacaine is also available with epinephrine, typically as a solution of 0.5% bupivacaine with 1:200,000 (0.005 mg/mL) epinephrine. It is hepatically metabolized. The maximum dose, with regard to systemic toxicity, is 2.5 mg/kg, not to exceed 175 mg per dose or 400 mg per 24 hours. Bupivacaine may provide supplemental analgesic effects by binding to the prostaglandin E2 receptor, reducing the production of prostaglandins and thereby reducing inflammation and hyperalgesia.

Ropivacaine is also an amide local anesthetic related structurally to bupivacaine.[18] It is the pure S(-) enantiomer of the racemic bupivacaine. It is typically produced as a ropivacaine hydrochloride salt. Ropivacaine is metabolized by the liver by aromatic hydroxylation via the cytochrome P450 system. The maximum dose, with regard to systemic toxicity, is 3 mg/kg, not to exceed 225 mg per dose.

As a class, local amide anesthetics affect all nerve fiber types. Thus, when they interact with the nerve trunk they can inhibit both sensory and motor fibers. Their effect, however, depends on the diameter, myelination, and conduction velocity of the fibers. Clinically, the nerve functions affected are as follows (from first to last affected): pain, temperature, touch, proprioception, muscle tone. As a class, the toxicity of local amide anesthetics can be lethal, primarily affecting the central nervous (CNS) and cardiovascular (CV) systems. Typically, CNS side effects occur at lower plasma concentrations than do CV side effects. Generalized CNS excitation (tingling at the mouth, tinnitus, blurred vision, seizures) occurs prior to generalized CNS depression (drowsiness, loss of consciousness, respiratory depression). The CV side effects may occur secondary to or independently of CNS side effects and include hypotension, bradycardia, arrhythmia, and cardiac arrest.

Treatment of local anesthetic systemic toxicity (LAST) depends on prompt recognition of the syndrome and halting administration of the offending agent. All local anesthetics can cause LAST, though differences in anesthetic potency correlate to the likelihood of cardiac toxicity (e.g., bupivacaine is more cardiotoxic than lidocaine). Ropivacaine, the pure S-enantiomer of bupivacaine, is less cardiotoxic and causes fewer CNS side effects. The doses required to cause cardiovascular collapse (CC) and CNS side effects can be compared in a ratio (CC:CNS), which theoretically describes the safety of local anesthetics with regard to serious adverse events (i.e., larger ratios correspond to a wider gap between doses that cause clinically recognizable CNS effects and life-threatening cardiovascular collapse). Among the anesthetics commonly used for SIJ procedures, bupivacaine has the lowest CC:CNS ratio in animal models, followed by ropivacaine, then lidocaine.

Treatment of LAST is described in guidelines and checklists published by the American Society of Regional Anesthesia and Pain Management. First steps include stopping any ongoing local anesthetic injection/infusion, calling for help, and early arrangement of cardiopulmonary bypass at the nearest facility. Managing the airway is the next step, including the administration of oxygen. If needed, endotracheal intubation should be performed with the goal of preventing acidosis, hypoxemia, and hypercarbia. Seizure suppression is vital as seizures may potentiate LAST. Intravenous benzodiazepine (e.g., midazolam 1–2 mg) is preferred to propofol to treat seizures, as the latter may exacerbate CC. In addition to advanced cardiac life support (ACLS) protocols, lipid emulsification (20%) should be administered at the following doses:

- For patients weighing less than 70 kg: bolus with 1.5 mL/kg given intravenously (IV), followed by infusion at 0.25 mL/kg/minute IV.
- For patients weighing more than 70 kg: 100 mL IV, followed by infusion of 200 to 250 mL IV over 15 to 20 minutes.

Management of cardiac effects, including arrhythmia and arrest, is different for LAST than other arrest scenarios, as prolonged quality compressions may be necessary to circulate lipid emulsifications. If there are persistent signs of CC, the bolus dose should be repeated one or two times with a maximum dose of about 12 mL/kg. Once the patient's cardiovascular status is stable, the infusion should continue for 10 minutes and the patient should be transferred to a monitored setting.

Despite their hepatic metabolism, the drug labels for amide anesthetics do not mention liver toxicity. Nevertheless, several case reports and case series have described liver toxicity with their use.[19] In general, to minimize the risk of these and other adverse events, the minimal necessary dose should be used in any form of anesthesia.

MAC

According to the American Society of Anesthesiologists (ASA), MAC is a specific service providing sedation and analgesia, titrated to keep patients comfortable but preserve spontaneous breathing and airway reflexes. It is used in 10% to 30% of all surgical procedures.[20] Use of MAC depends on the level of consciousness/sedation required for the procedure as well as accessibility of the airway in the event that general anesthesia is required. General anesthesia is better suited in procedures that necessitate deeper sedation or limit access to the airway, or in patients at high risk for aspiration. MAC typically involves the use of a variety of sedatives and pain medications given intravenously. Drug choice is dependent on the provider.

In the context of SIJ procedures, MAC is typically seen with the Simplicity RFA technique and minimally invasive joint fusions. In Simplicity RFA, MAC allows for painless placement of the probe as well as sufficient sedation for the ablation itself. Minimally invasive SIJ fusion has been used in refractory SIJ pain. In theory, a relatively small amount of movement of the pathologic joint can cause low back pain, and this may be reduced/eliminated by fusing the joint. There are multiple minimally invasive SIJ fusion techniques. Postprocedural local anesthesia is usually provided in addition to MAC in these cases.

During procedures using MAC, standard ASA monitoring procedures (temperature, pulse oximetry, blood pressure and heart rate, electrocardiogram) should be employed. Capnography (exhaled CO_2 monitoring) should also be used, as it may serve as a portent of apnea or airway obstruction. Electroencephalography has been described to monitor the depth of sedation in MAC but is not routinely used for SIJ cases in our experience. Clinical monitoring, as per the ASA definitions of minimal, moderate, and deep sedation, should be employed throughout these procedures to evaluate patient arousability and to avoid general anesthesia. Supplemental oxygen is not necessary with MAC, particularly if minimal sedation is used and the patient has no significant cardiovascular risk factors. If moderate or deep sedation is achieved, supplemental oxygen is generally required.

The most common serious side effects of MAC as reported by the ASA are respiratory in nature: airway obstruction, respiratory depression, and aspiration. Cardiovascular compromise and local anestheticsystemic toxicity are also possible serious adverse events. Among the drugs used for MAC, the most common include midazolam, propofol, opioids, dexmedetomidine, and ketamine.

Midazolam

Midazolam is a short-acting benzodiazepine and shares the effect of other drugs in this class, including anxiety reduction and amnesia without analgesia. The onset of action with IV administration is 1 to 3 minutes and the duration of action is 1 to 4 hours. An initial dose of 0.5 to 2 mg IV can be given both in the preoperative area and prior to administration of propofol in the operating room. The dose should be reduced in the elderly. It is important to note that midazolam potentiates the effects of other opiates, with the substantial risk of respiratory depression. Flumazenil is a benzodiazepine antagonist that can be used to reverse the sedation of midazolam but does not reverse the respiratory depression of opiates. The initial dose of flumazenil is 0.2 mg IV given over 15 seconds, with repeated doses every 1 minute up to a maximum dose of 1 mg. This pattern can be repeated every 20 minutes if needed.

Propofol

Propofol is a hypnotic/sedative with antiemetic and moderate amnestic effects, commonly used in surgical procedures due to its favorable pharmacokinetic profile. Its short elimination half-life allows for rapid patient recovery from sedation if necessary. It can be administered IV as a bolus (about 20 mg) or as a continuous titration (usually 25–75 mcg/kg/minute). There is a narrow therapeutic index and no reversal agent, so patients must be monitored carefully for oversedation and airway compromise. Pretreatment with injected lidocaine and use of large veins may prevent the pain associated with propofol injection.

Opioids

Opioids may be used in MAC for analgesia, supplementing the sedation provided by other agents. Fentanyl and remifentanil are commonly used. Postoperative nausea and vomiting associated with opiate use should be treated prophylactically if propofol is not being used for MAC. Fentanyl is typically administered in intermittent 25- to 50-microgram IV doses. The onset is anywhere from 1 to 3 minutes and the duration of action ranges from 30 to 60 minutes. Remifentanil has an onset of action of 60 to 90 seconds and an elimination half-life of 3 minutes. Dosing depends on a multitude of patient factors as well as the concomitant use of midazolam.

Dexmedetomidine

Dexmedetomidine is an alpha-2 adrenergic agonist with sedative, anxiolytic, and analgesic effects. The loading dose is 0.5 to 1.0 mcg/kg over 10 minutes. The infusion rate is usually 0.2 to 1.0 mcg/kg/hour. The onset time is approximately 15 minutes after a loading dose. Elimination half-lives vary with infusion durations, varying from 4 to 250 minutes. However, the slow onset, long duration of action, and cardiovascular effects make dexmedetomidine less than ideal for SIJ procedures.

Ketamine

Ketamine is a sedative with amnestic and analgesic effects in part due to NMDA-receptor antagonism. It is often given preoperatively since it has been shown to reduce postoperative opioid dose requirements. The dose is 0.25 to 0.5 mg/kg IV. The onset is rapid, about 1 minute. The duration of action is 20 to 30 minutes and the elimination half-life is 2 to 3 hours. Side effects vary from heart rate and blood pressure elevations to cardiovascular depression in patients with catecholamine deficits. Increased oral secretions, laryngospasm, and hallucinations can occur as well but are less likely at the recommended 0.25- to 0.5-mg/kg doses.

Neuraxial anesthesia

Neuraxial anesthesia involves the injection of anesthetics between the vertebrae into either the subarachnoid or epidural space. It is most commonly performed for procedures of the lower limbs or lower abdomen. In the context of SIJ procedures, spinal anesthesia, via epidural or intrathecal routes, may be considered in cases of minimally invasive SIJ fusions. Minimally invasive SIJ fusion is based on the same concept as invasive fusions—that is, that pain relief can be achieved by stopping the small degree of motion that naturally occurs at the junction of the pelvis and the sacrum. It is more commonly described via a lateral approach, and there are data supporting its use dating back to at least 2008.[7,21] Multiple fusion systems exist and a detailed description of each is beyond the scope of this text. However, it should be noted that in multiple studies, general anesthesia was the preferred form of anesthesia for these minimally invasive SIJ fusions.

Neuraxial anesthesia can be divided into three distinct types: spinal (i.e., intrathecal or subarachnoid), epidural, and combined spinal and epidural (CSE). Spinal anesthesia is most commonly performed at the L3–4 or the L4–5 interspace. Higher vertebral levels of injection may risk injury to the spinal cord, which usually terminates at the caudal aspect of the first lumbar vertebral body. Lower injection sites such as the L5–S1 interspace may require larger volumes to reach the thoracic nerve roots, which may require anesthesia in some spinal surgeries. The target of the spinal block is the subarachnoid space (between the pia and arachnoid mater) wherein the cerebrospinal fluid (CSF) sits along with the spinal nerves and blood vessels. The spinal level refers to the most rostral level anesthetized by a spinal block. Of note, autonomic fibers are affected by spinal blocks. In particular, given the level of the injection, the splanchnic parasympathetic roots of S2–4 are preferentially blocked compared to the sympathetic nerve roots originating between T1 and L2. Blocks are generally performed in the sitting, lateral decubitus, or prone position. Small-diameter (24 to 27 gauge), pencil-point needles are preferred given a lower propensity to cause post-dural puncture headache (PDPH). PDPH is a common side effect of spinal blocks in addition to the more short-term side effects of hypotension, urinary retention, and motor weakness. An epidural block, in contrast, does not require a dural puncture, thereby reducing the risk of PDPH. Epidural injections also have the benefit of continuous injections, including injection in the postoperative phase of care. Injection into the epidural space carries a longer onset time compared to a spinal block. A CSE block provides both the rapid onset of action of the spinal block and the prolonged duration of action of the epidural block. However, a combined block takes longer to perform than a single spinal block injection. Furthermore, confirmation of a functioning epidural catheter is complicated by preceding spinal injection. Ultimately the choice among these three types of neuraxial anesthesia for minimally invasive SIJ fusions depends on the practitioner.

Baricity is an important concept with regard to neuraxial anesthesia and drug choice. Baricity refers to the relative density of anesthetic solutions to the density of CSF. In a double-blind study of bupivacaine solutions with different densities, hyperbaric bupivacaine was shown to provide higher spinal levels compared to isobaric or hypobaric bupivacaine.[22,23] Bupivacaine, the most commonly used anesthetic in spinal blocks, can be made hyperbaric by the addition of dextrose and hypobaric by the addition of sterile water. Doses used for bupivacaine in spinal blocks range from 6 to 15 mg, with a duration of action of 1 to 2 hours. Lidocaine has become less popular for spinal blocks given the higher rate of short-term neurologic side effects. However, its shorter duration of action makes it a reasonable choice in ambulatory settings. Doses range from 40 to 100 mg, with a duration of 45 to 75 minutes. Use of ropivacaine is more common outside of the United States and may confer less of a motor block compared to the closely related racemic bupivacaine. Doses of ropivacaine used for spinal blocks range from 15 to 20 mg and have a duration of action of 75 to 120 minutes. Opioids and alpha-adrenergic agonists can be combined with anesthetics at the discretion of the provider.

General anesthesia

General anesthesia is the most sedating and oldest form of anesthesia. sIt was originally described in 1842 by Crawford Long using diethyl ether. Since then, advances in pharmacology and patient care have substantially improved outcomes and increased the complexity of general anesthesia. Some concepts outlined here may be important for SIJ procedures. Lateral fusions as described in the prior section may benefit from general anesthesia, if there are contraindications to neuraxial anesthesia or based on provider preference. Open SIJ fusions will usually require general anesthesia.

Classically, there are four stages of anesthesia: (1) analgesia (conscious), (2) delirium (unconscious, irregular breathing), (3) surgical anesthesia (unable to protect airway), and (4) respiratory arrest (medullary depression) (Table 5.3). The goal of general anesthesia is to induce a reversible state of stage 3 anesthesia. It is suitable for most surgeries. General anesthesia may be divided into the induction, maintenance, and emergence phases.

Induction

Induction is typically achieved with a combination of a sedative, an adjunctive agent (opioid, amide anesthetic, or benzodiazepine), and a neuromuscular blocking agent. Sedatives commonly used include propofol, ketamine, or etomidate. Propofol is typically dosed at 1 to 2.5 mg/kg, etomidate at 0.15 to 0.3 mg/kg, and ketamine at 1 to 2 mg/kg. Adjuncts like fentanyl are dosed at 0.5 to 1 mcg/kg (or commonly 25–100 mcg), sufentanil at 0.05 to 0.1 mcg/kg, lidocaine at 0.5 to 1.5 mg/kg, and midazolam at 1-mg increments up to 4 mg. Please note these doses may need reduction in elderly and hemodynamically unstable patients. A number of neuromuscular blocks agents are available. Succinylcholine is often used due to its rapid onset of action (about 1 minute) and ultrashort duration of action. The intubating dose of succinylcholine is 0.6 to 1.5 mg/kg. The elimination half-life is less than 1 minute. After induction, placement of an endotracheal tube with the distal end in the trachea is the most commonly used airway device for general anesthesia. Supraglottic airway (SGA) devices, most commonly a laryngeal mask airway (LMA), may be used as a rescue device in cases of difficult intubations. However, SGA devices do not block the pharynx and therefore may cause gastric insufflation and/or hypoventilation. To reduce this risk, pressure-control (or pressure-limited) ventilation is preferred with SGA devices as opposed to volume-control ventilation.

Maintenance

Maintenance of general anesthesia is achieved with inhaled anesthetics and IV sedatives. The goal of using multiple drugs is to take advantage of their synergistic effects to achieve stage 3 anesthesia while limiting the total dose of any one drug. The inhaled anesthetics

TABLE 5.3 Stages of anesthesia

Stage 1	Analgesia	Conscious
Stage 2	Delirium	Unconscious, irregular breathing
Stage 3	Surgical anesthesia	Unconscious, unable to protect airway
Stage 4	Medullary depression	Unconscious, respiratory arrest

include nitrous oxide, halothane, isoflurane, sevoflurane, and desflurane. Dosing is dependent on age, coexisting conditions, and coadministration with other anesthetics. Total intravenous anesthesia (TIVA) does not use any inhaled anesthetic; instead, IV propofol (due to its rapid onset and recovery, antiemetic properties, and generally benign side-effect profile) is typically used with an opioid adjuvant. If near-complete muscle relaxation is required, a neuromuscular blocking agent may be employed.

Emergence

Emergence from general anesthesia is typically a passive process. If neuromuscular blocking agents are used, assessing their effect and reversal is necessary. If an endotracheal tube was placed, several extubation techniques are available, including the standard low-risk extubation, deep extubation, and the remifentanil extubation technique. Transporting the patient to the post-anesthesia care unit can be safely performed once patients are ventilating spontaneously, oxygenating adequately, responding appropriately to commands, and hemodynamically stable.

Conclusion

The purpose of this chapter is to provide an overview of the anesthetic techniques commonly used in the context of SIJ procedures (Table 5.4). These discussions should provide practitioners a guide to choosing the most appropriate anesthesia for common SIJ procedures. Common concepts, such as using the lowest effective doses of the drugs discussed, apply across these different techniques. More specific concepts, such as the effect of pKa, lipophilicity, and protein binding on amide anesthetic properties, as well as baricity in spinal anesthesia, are important clinically and suggest the complexity of anesthetic physiology and

TABLE 5.4 SIJ procedures and recommended levels of anesthesia

Procedure	Anesthesia	Injectate
Diagnostic SIJ injection	None	1% lidocaine
Therapeutic SIJ injection	Local anesthesia w/ 3–5 cc 1% lidocaine	Bupivacaine or ropivacaine ± corticosteroid
SIJ nerve block	Local anesthesia w/ 3–5 cc 1% lidocaine	Bupivacaine or ropivacaine
SIJ nerve ablation	Local anesthesia w/ 3–5 cc 1% lidocaine	N/A
Simplicity SIJ nerve ablation	MAC (midazolam, propofol, opioids, dexmedetomidine, ketamine; see text for dosing)	N/A
Minimally invasive SIJ Fusion	MAC vs. neuraxial vs. general anesthesia	N/A
Open SIJ fusion	General anesthesia	N/A

pharmacology. To further explore these concepts and for more detailed information on these techniques, the reader is directed to primary anesthesia literature.

References

1. Skaribas IM, et al. Sacroiliac joint injection. In TR Deer, et al. (Eds.), *Deer's treatment of pain: An illustrated guide for practitioners* (pp. 429–432). Springer International Publishing, 2019. doi:10.1007/978-3-030-12281-2_52

2. Chou LH, et al. Inciting events initiating injection-proven sacroiliac joint syndrome. *Pain Med.* 2004;5(1):26–32. doi:10.1111/j.1526-4637.2004.04009.x

3. Fortin JD, et al. Sacroiliac joint: Pain referral maps upon applying a new injection/arthrography technique. Part I: Asymptomatic volunteers. *Spine*. 1994;19:1475–1482.

4. Poilliot AJ, et al. A systematic review of the normal sacroiliac joint anatomy and adjacent tissues for pain physicians. *Pain Physician*. 2019;22(4):E247–E274.

5. Hammonds WD, Steinhaus JE. Crawford W. Long: Pioneer physician in anesthesia. *J Clin Anesth.* 1993;5(2):163–167. doi:10.1016/0952-8180(93)90147-7

6. Connor H, Connor T. Did the use of chloroform by Queen Victoria influence its acceptance in obstetric practice? *Anaesthesia*. 1996;51(10):955–957, doi:10.1111/j.1365-2044.1996.tb14964.x

7. Al-Khayer A, et al. Percutaneous sacroiliac joint arthrodesis: A novel technique. *J Spinal Disord Tech.* 2008;21(5):359–363.

8. American Society of Anesthesiologists Task Force on Chronic Pain Management and the American Society of Regional Anesthesia and Pain Medicine. Practice guidelines for chronic pain management: An updated report. *Anesthesiology*. 2010;112(4):810–833, doi:10.1097/ALN.0b013e3181c43103

9. Zheng P, et al. Image-guided sacroiliac joint injections: An evidence-based review of best practices and clinical outcomes. *PM & R*. 2019;11(Suppl. 1):S98–S104. doi:10.1002/pmrj.12191

10. Chen AS, et al. Procedural pain during lumbar medial branch blocks with and without skin wheal anesthesia: A prospective comparative observational study. *Pain Med.* 2019;20(4):779–783. doi:10.1093/pm/pny322

11. Ackerman WE, et al. Are diagnostic lumbar facet injections influenced by pain of muscular origin? *Pain Practice*. 2004;4(4):286–291. doi:10.1111/j.1533-2500.2004.04402.x

12. Cohen SP, et al. Facet joint pain: Advances in patient selection and treatment. *Nature Rev Rheumatol.* 2013;9(2):101–116. doi:10.1038/nrrheum.2012.198

13. Griffith RJ, et al. Vapocoolants (cold spray) for pain treatment during intravenous cannulation. *Cochrane Database Syst Rev.* 2016;4:CD009484. doi:10.1002/14651858.CD009484.pub2

14. Hogan M-E, et al. Systematic review and meta-analysis of the effect of warming local anesthetics on injection pain. *Ann Emerg Med.* 2011;58(1):86–98. doi:10.1016/j.annemergmed.2010.12.001

15. Guo J, et al. Efficacy of sodium bicarbonate buffered versus non-buffered lidocaine with epinephrine in inferior alveolar nerve block: A meta-analysis. *J Dent Anesth Pain Med.* 2018;18(3):129–142. doi:10.17245/jdapm.2018.18.3.129

16. National Center for Biotechnology Information. PubChem Database. Lidocaine, CID=3676. https://pubchem.ncbi.nlm.nih.gov/compound/Lidocaine

17. National Center for Biotechnology Information. PubChem Database. Bupivacaine, CID=2474. https://pubchem.ncbi.nlm.nih.gov/compound/Bupivacaine

18. National Center for Biotechnology Information. PubChem Database. Ropivacaine, CID=175805. https://pubchem.ncbi.nlm.nih.gov/compound/Ropivacaine

19. Chintamaneni P, et al. Bupivacaine drug-induced liver injury: A case series and brief review of the literature. *J Clin Anesth.* 2016;32:137–141. doi:10.1016/j.jclinane.2016.01.035

20. Das S, Ghosh S. Monitored anesthesia care: An overview. *J Anaesthesiol Clin Pharmacol.* 2015;31(1):27–29. doi:10.4103/0970-9185.150525

22. Wise CL, Dall BE. Minimally invasive sacroiliac arthrodesis: Outcomes of a new technique. *J Spinal Disord Tech.* 2008;21(8):579–584.

23. Chambers WA, et al. Effect of baricity on spinal anaesthesia with bupivacaine. *Br J Anaesth.* 1981;53(3):279–282. doi:10.1093/bja/53.3.279

PART II

Sacroiliac joint interventions

6

Intraarticular injections (ultrasound-guided and fluoroscopic-guided approaches)

Luay Mrad, Akshat Gargya, and Rany T. Abdallah

Introduction

Sacroiliac joint (SIJ) pain has long been recognized as a potential source of chronic low back pain. Its prevalence is estimated to be about 15% to 30% in patients who present with chronic low back pain.[1,2] SIJ pain is implicated in up to 40% of patients with new-onset low back pain after lumbar arthrodesis.[3] Pain from SIJ can mimic several other conditions and needs to be differentiated by proper history and physical examination. These conditions most commonly include a herniated disc or hip joint pathology. The SIJ is a synovial joint filled with fluid. The joint derives its innervations mainly from the dorsal rami of sacral nerves. This joint can be affected in multiple inflammatory processes such as ankylosing spondylitis and rheumatoid arthritis. Other common causes of SIJ dysfunction and pain include trauma and osteoarthritis.

Symptoms of SIJ dysfunction involve lower back and buttock pain that may radiate to the hip and upper thigh area. Symptoms are usually worse with physical activities like walking, moving from sitting to standing position, sleeping, or sitting on the affected side. Although no diagnostic criteria consensus has been established to diagnose SIJ pain, diagnosis usually starts with obtaining a detailed history and physical examination. Multiple provocative maneuvers have been described in the past, such as the Fortin finger sign and the flexion abduction external rotation (FABER) test (see Chapter 3). Imaging such as X-ray, magnetic resonance imaging (MRI), or computed tomography (CT) scanning may provide additional support in establishing an accurate diagnosis and ruling out other potential causes of low back pain.[4]

First-line treatment in SIJ dysfunction usually involves conservative management such as physical therapy, stretching exercises, nonsteroidal anti-inflammatory drugs (NSAIDs), and local topical patches/creams. In cases of failed conservative management, intraarticular steroid injection in the joint is performed using fluoroscopy or ultrasound guidance. The third line of treatment usually involves SIJ radiofrequency ablation or SIJ fusion, which could provide longer relief and a better outcome in addition to avoiding long-term use of steroids.

The effectiveness of nonsurgical treatments for chronic SIJ pain remains unclear. Periarticular radiofrequency ablation and intraarticular corticosteroid injections are supported only by short-term evidence. From our clinical practice, SIJ intraarticular injection is usually effective in reducing pain for 3 to 4 months and provides moderate to significant relief. Radiofrequency ablation has been shown to provide longer relief that usually lasts anywhere from 6 to 12 months. Surgical arthrodesis of the SIJ remains an option if all other treatment approaches have failed.

Fluoroscopy-guided SIJ injection technique

Fluoroscopy-guided SIJ injection can be performed in a dedicated procedure room or operating room. The patient is prepped in sterile fashion and is placed in a prone position. A pillow may be placed under the abdomen at the level of the iliac crests. To visualize the inferior portion of the SIJ, the C-arm is initially placed in anterior–posterior (AP) view and then moved to a contralateral oblique view for optimal visualization of the joint line. At this point, the C-arm can also be tilted cranially or caudally to allow for better visualization of the inferior aspect of the joint. When the bony planes of the inferior portion of the joints are parallel, the image is considered ideal.

The identified area is then marked. The superficial skin and subcutaneous tissues are then anesthetized using 1% or 2% lidocaine. With intermittent fluoroscopy, the 22-gauge spinal needle is advanced in a coaxial manner to the inferior part of the SIJ. Once the needle reaches the joint, a distinct popping sensation can be felt by the physician when the needle traverses inside the joint space. To confirm the depth of the needle, a lateral image is recommended at this point. Care must be taken to make sure the needle does not traverse the joint cavity, as there are case reports of inadvertent sciatic nerve injury. Contrast (0.5 cc) is now injected to confirm the needle placement (Figure 6.1). Once optimal needle position is achieved within the inferior portion of the SIJ, a combination of local anesthetic and steroid is injected into the joint space. We recommend using at least 20 to 40 mg triamcinolone along with 1 to 2 cc 0.25% to 5% bupivacaine. However, a recent study done by Nacey et al. showed that periarticular SIJ injection can provide similar significant reduction in pain when compared to intraarticular SIJ injection.[5]

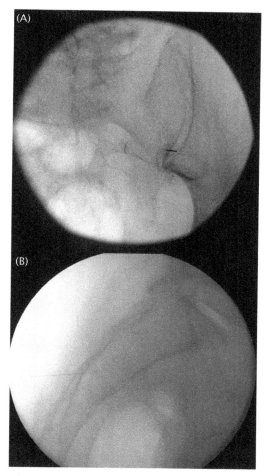

FIGURE 6.1. Anteroposterior (**A**) and lateral (**B**) images of fluoroscopic-guided SIJ injection.

Ultrasound-guided SIJ injection technique

Ultrasound-guided SIJ injection is preferred in pregnant patients to avoid exposure and risk of complications from radiation. Ultrasound is also beneficial in avoiding vascular injury, as shown by a recent randomized prospective study.[6] This imaging modality, however, has less accuracy than fluoroscopy.[6]

To successfully perform an ultrasound-guided SIJ injection, the patient is placed in a prone position. A curvilinear transducer probe is recommended since it can cover a wider area under the probe and is also effective in finding the joint in obese patients. A cushion or bolster may be placed under the patient's pelvis to facilitate SIJ opening. Musculoskeletal settings on the ultrasound machine are recommended to better visualize and enhance the bony structures under ultrasound.

Under strict aseptic conditions, the ultrasound probe is first placed in the transverse position to find the base of the sacrum. This can be facilitated by finding the anatomic midline by identifying the spinous process of the lumbar vertebra and then scanning caudally to locate the top of the sacrum. The probe is then moved laterally and caudally to identify the posterior-superior iliac spine (PSIS). Just medial and caudal to the PSIS, a hypoechoic shadow cast by the iliac crest can then be seen between the PSIS and the sacrum. This potential space is the SIJ. The skin is then anesthetized with 1% or 2% lidocaine. With the use of an in-plane technique, a 25G 3.5- to 5-inch spinal needle or a 21G 4-inch echogenic ultrasound needle is inserted in a medial to lateral trajectory toward the SIJ (Figure 6.2). Once the needle reaches the SIJ, the syringe is aspirated to rule out intravascular spread. If aspiration is negative, a solution containing local anesthetic and steroid can then be injected

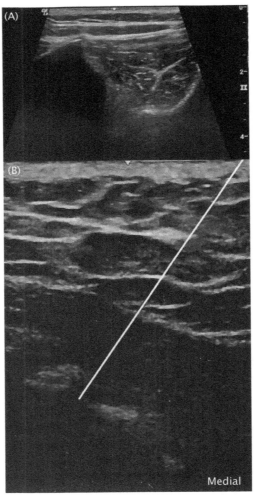

FIGURE 6.2. (**A**) Ultrasound images showing wide-angle SIJ. (**B**) Closeup angle with the needle directed to the SIJ.

in the joint. We recommend using at least 20 to 40 mg triamcinolone along with 1 to 2 cc 0.25% to 0.5% bupivacaine.

References

1. Bernard TN, Jr, Kirkaldy-Willis WH. Recognizing specific characteristics of nonspecific low back pain. Clin Orthop Relat Res. 1987;217:266–280.
2. Schwarzer AC, Aprill CN, Bogduk N. The sacroiliac joint in chronic low back pain. Spine (Phila Pa 1976). 1995;20(1):31–37.
3. DePalma MJ, Ketchum JM, Saullo T. What is the source of chronic low back pain and does the age play a role? Pain Med. 2011;12:224–233.
4. Tuite M. Sacroiliac joint imaging. Semin Musculoskel Radiol. 2008;12(1):72–82.
5. Nacey N, Patrie J, Fox M. Fluoroscopically guided sacroiliac joint injections: Comparison of the effects of intraarticular and periarticular injections on immediate and short-term pain relief. AJR Am J Roentgenol. 2016;207(5):1055–1061.
6. Jee H, Lee J, Park K, Ahn J, Park Y. Ultrasound-guided versus fluoroscopy guided sacroiliac joint intra-articular injections in the noninflammatory sacroiliac joint dysfunction: A prospective, randomized, single-blinded study. Arch Phys Med Rehab. 2014;95(2):330–337.

7

Lateral branch blocks

Benjamin K. Homra, Yashar Eshraghi, and Maged Guirguis

Introduction

The complex innervation of the sacroiliac joint (SIJ) has traditionally made intraarticular injections the preferred therapeutic modality for SIJ pain. However, the increased use of radiofrequency ablation (RFA) targeting the posterior joint has highlighted the need for diagnostic blocks of those nerves. The exact innervation of the joint is contentious, with some believing the joint is supplied by both an anterior and posterior source and others suggesting it is exclusively posterior.[1] The consensus is that the SIJ derives its innervation from the L4 and L5 posterior primary rami and the lateral branches of the S1–S3 dorsal rami.[2] Regardless of the belief that one holds, the sacral dorsal rami play a large role in the transmission of pain from the SIJ. Targeting this plexus of nerves with local anesthetic provides a diagnostic block that serves as a prognostic test for the success of RFA of the nerve. These lateral branch blocks (LBBs) will be the subject of this chapter.

Anatomic considerations

An understanding of the anatomy of the posterior sacral network (PSN) is important in targeting the lateral branches as they vary in terms of sacral level and position of emergence from the foramina. Prior to forming the PSN, the lateral branches derive from the spinal cord's terminus, located at the level of L1–L2 in adults, where it transitions into the cauda equina. The cauda equina is a bundle of spinal nerves that consists of the second through fifth lumbar nerve pairs, the first through fifth sacral nerve pairs, and the coccygeal nerve. The sacral nerves of the cauda equina travel from the conus medullaris down the lumbar spinal canal and emerge from the sacral canal through both the anterior and posterior (dorsal) sacral foramina and become anterior and dorsal rami.

The anterior rami predominantly form the sacral plexus, which provides motor and sensory nerves for the posterior thigh, most of the lower leg and foot, and part of the pelvis. The anterior innervation of the SIJ is beyond the scope of this chapter, but there is debate

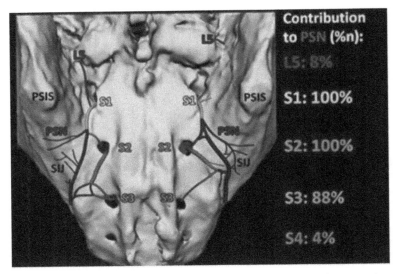

FIGURE 7.1. Overview of the innervation of the SIJ, posterolateral view with percent innervation to the PSN.

as to whether the anterior rami innervate the SIJ at all. The consensus appears to be that nerve filaments from L4–S2 may supply the ventral SIJ based on cadaveric studies.[3] This is less clinically relevant as the majority of the joint's innervation stems from the dorsal rami's lateral branches, while the anterior branches are difficult to target through vital organs and carry a high risk of neuropathy due to their relationship with the sacral plexus.

The lateral branches of the sacrum are terminal filaments of the sacral dorsal rami that form the PSN from multiple sacral (and lumbar) levels and innervate the dorsal SIJ. Regarding the level, cadaveric studies show that that the S1 and S2 lateral branches contribute to the PSN in 100% of specimens, S3 in 77%, L5 in 8%, and S4 in 4% (Figure 7.1).[4] While the S1–S3 dorsal rami contribute most consistently to the PSN, the number of lateral branches emerging from each level varied. Again, cadaveric studies concluded that these branches exited from the 2- to 6-o'clock position on the right or the 6- to 10-o'clock position on the left.[4] Ultimately, the lateral branches contributing to the PSN cross the lateral sacral crest between the first and the third transverse sacral tubercle.

Now that the proceduralist is equipped with a theoretical understanding of the PSN's anatomy, he or she now needs to choose the method by which to reach the target. An LBB can be performed under fluoroscopic or ultrasound guidance. The technique, advantages, and disadvantages will be addressed in the next sections.

Fluoroscopic guidance

Soto et al. describe a multisite, multi-depth 16-injection technique under fluoroscopy.[5] The patient is placed prone, and imaging is then obtained at the L5–S1 disk space. Sedation is discouraged to limit confounding pain relief from intravenous medications. Using a high-concentration, long-acting local anesthetic like 0.75% bupivacaine provides up to 24 hours' worth of potential relief and allows ample time for patients to perform their daily activities and encounter typical pain generators. Use of steroids or other additives should be discouraged in order to accurately assess the LBB's efficacy. Spinal needles are placed peripherally above the posterior sacral foramina at 8 to 10 mm. The sacral foramina should be thought of as a clockface, with the lateral margin being the center of the face. On the right side, at the S1 and S2 levels, the needles are placed at the 2:30, 4:00, and 5:30 positions. At the same levels on the left, needles are placed at 9:30, 8:00, and 6:30 positions. At the S3 level, needles are placed at 2:30 and 4:00 on the right and 9:30 and 8:00 on the left. Each of these targets is then injected with 0.2 mL 0.75% bupivacaine, the needle is pulled back approximately 3 mm, and another 0.2 mL bupivacaine is injected. This method was studied in a randomized control study compared to injecting placebo. Dreyfuss et al. found that seven of the 10 patients in the local anesthetic arm reported a significant decrease in pain from repeat probing of the foraminal ligaments, while only one of the 10 patients in the placebo arm reported pain relief on repeat probing.[1] However, only two of the 10 patients in the local anesthetic arm and zero of the 10 patients in the placebo arm were protected from pain on repeat stimulation of the intraarticular joint.

This multisite, multi-depth technique serves to maximize the area that the lateral branches typically course through.[2] The lateral branches do not run in a constant plane; they may be located superficially or deep to the posterior sacroiliac ligament. Therefore, a needle placed on the dorsal surface of the sacrum would fail to anesthetize the target nerve if it runs more superficially above the posterior sacroiliac ligament. Local anesthetic placed at two depths takes into account the various planes of the lateral branches' course. Additionally, the lateral branches do not emerge from the posterior sacral foramina at a consistent location; as previously mentioned, cadaveric studies demonstrated that lateral branches may radiate cephalad, transversely, or caudad. Injecting at multiple sites using a clockface as a reference point will maximize the ability to cover the likely point of emergence (Figure 7.2).

Ultrasound guidance

For the ultrasound-guided LBB technique, the patient is positioned prone with the sacrum scanned on the transverse plane. As with the fluoroscopic technique, IV sedation, steroids, or additives should be discouraged and a high-concentration, long-acting local anesthetic should be used. A C5-2 MHz curved transducer is placed on the lower sacrum and the sacral hiatus is identified, which signifies the midline.[6] The probe is then moved laterally to the target site while keeping the median sacral crest in view. The probe should then be moved cephalad to visualize the posterior sacral foramina and the lateral sacral crest. For this block, the lateral sacral crest is the target—specifically between the S2 and S3 transverse tubercle, immediately above the S2 transverse tubercle, and at the level of the S1 tubercle directly. An in-plane needle technique is used to inject local anesthetic at these three target sites: 1.5 mL between S2 and S3, 0.5 mL immediately above S2, and 0.5

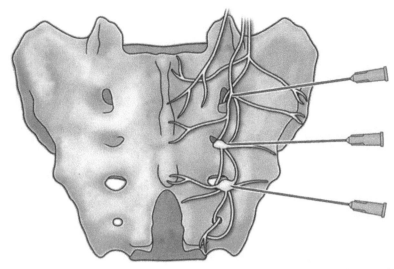

FIGURE 7.2. Lateral branches from S1 to S4 sacral foramen. Schematic drawing showing the S1–3 lateral branches innervating the SIJ and overlying ligaments. The needles depict the approximate location for the diagnostic LBB.

mL lateral to S1 (Figure 7.3).[7] Prior to injection, a sagittal scan is performed to confirm needle placement in the cephalocaudal dimension. The posterior foramina will appear as gaps in the hyperechoic bony contour of the sacrum. This aptly named triple-target technique is the more favorable ultrasound-guided block. Attempts have been made to use a one-injection technique at the S2 level, but local anesthetic has not reliably spread to the S1 level.[8] The double-injection technique (below S2 and at the S1 level) needs further validation.

Comparison of techniques

There is one randomized controlled trial that compared the two modalities, with procedure duration being the primary endpoint.[7] The procedure performed using the ultrasound technique was significantly shorter than the one using the fluoroscopic technique. However, the procedure times varied with the level of expertise under ultrasound but were similar under fluoroscopy. Interestingly, the block efficacy showed no difference between the two techniques, despite more specific targeting of the PSN under fluoroscopy.

Risks and contraindications

Both the fluoroscopy- and ultrasound-guided LBBs are considered safe procedures with minimal risks and contraindications. As with most interventional pain procedures, the risks of bleeding and infection are minimal but remain the most commonly encountered adverse events. The American Society of Regional Anesthesia and Pain Medicine considers

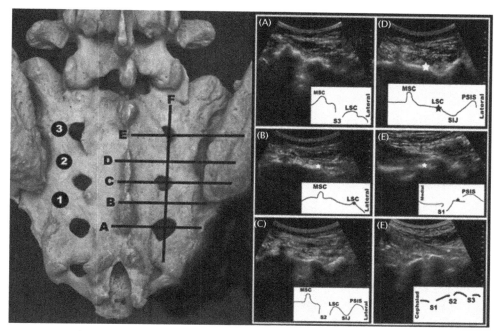

FIGURE 7.3. (Left) Posterior view of the sacrum on a skeletal model. Left side of the model depicts the injection points for an ultrasound-guided sacral LBB on the lateral sacral crest between the S2 and S3 transverse sacral tubercles (1); on the lateral crest immediately above the S2 transverse sacral tubercle (2); and on the lateral crest at the level of the S1 transverse sacral tubercle (3). Right side of the model depicts the individual scan lines corresponding to the sonograms on the right side of the figure. **(Right)** Sonographic images of the posterior sacrum depicting the various views required for the performance of an ultrasound-guided sacral LBB. This view is used to confirm needle positions prior to injection (biplanar technique). Injection points are marked by a star, and scan lines are illustrated on the left side of this figure. **(A)** Transverse sonographic view of the lower sacrum demonstrating the median sacral crest, posterior foramen of S3, and lateral sacral crest (LSC). **(B)** Transverse scan of the lower sacrum depicting the injection point on the LSC, at the midpoint between the posterior foramina of S3 and S2. **(C)** Transverse scan at the level of the S2 posterior foramen illustrating the caudad aspects of the SIJ and posterior superior iliac spine. **(D)** Transverse scan of the posterior sacrum demonstrating the injection point on the lateral sacral crest cephalad to the S2 posterior foramen. **(E)** Transverse scan of the sacrum illustrating the injection point lateral to the S1 posterior foramen. **(F)** Sagittal sonographic view of the sacrum with visualization of the posterior foramina of S1, S2, and S3. *Source:* Images used with permission by Finlayson RJ et al. (reference 7).

sacral LBBs to be peripheral nerve blocks and thus a low-risk procedure for a patient on antiplatelet or anticoagulant medication.[9] Therefore, current anticoagulant or antiplatelet medication use is not a contraindication for the block. The lateral branches are easily compressible, superficial nerves without major vascular structures in the vicinity of the block site. Therefore, in most situations, these medications do not need to be held prior to an LBB. The provider should remain cautious and ensure the patient has no other risk factors for bleeding. Regarding infection, these procedures should be performed using proper hand hygiene and sterile technique with gown and glove, and local anesthetic vials should not be reused. Injecting any local anesthetic always runs the risk of local anesthetic toxicity (LAST), and signs and symptoms should be monitored when administering high-concentration bupivacaine. The risk of LAST remains extremely low for LBBs due to the poor absorption of local anesthetic at the site and the small amount of bupivacaine used. For instance, a 75-kg patient's maximum dose of 0.75% bupivacaine would be 225 mg or 30 mL.

Implications

LBBs represent a diagnostic test and do not confer long-term relief of SIJ pain. Fortunately, it has been shown that subjects with confirmed SIJ pain who obtained 50% or greater pain relief from an LBB had a very high success rate of gaining long-term relief with RFA of those same nerves. Cohen et al. found that eight of their nine subjects who underwent RFA reported significant relief (50% or greater) after a successful LBB.[2] Failure to respond to LBBs could possibly arise for two reasons:

1. There is still considerable debate about the anterior innervation of the SIJ. If this is a large contributor to joint pain, then LBBs and RFAs would be ineffective in eliminating the pain signals relayed from those nerves.
2. The posterior innervation of the joint is variable and complex. Despite our knowledge of the anatomy and imaging techniques that visualize the targets, there is no guarantee that every nerve has been localized.

Overall, these techniques have proven to be of great benefit in temporarily treating SIJ pain and correlate well to successful RFA of the SIJ's posterior innervation.

References

1. Dreyfuss P, Henning T, Malladi N, Goldstein B, Bogduk N. The ability of multi-site, multi-depth sacral lateral branch blocks to anesthetize the sacroiliac joint complex. Pain Med. 2009;10(4):679–688. doi:10.1111/j.1526-4637.2009.00631.x. PMID: 19638143.
2. Cohen SP, Abdi S. Lateral branch blocks as a treatment for sacroiliac joint pain: A pilot study. Reg Anesth Pain Med. 2003;28(2):113–119. doi:10.1053/rapm.2003.50029. PMID: 12677621.
3. Bernard TN, Cassidy JD. The sacroiliac syndrome. Pathophysiology, diagnosis and management. In JW Frymoyer (Ed.), The adult spine: principles and practice (pp. 2107–2130). Raven, 1991.
4. Roberts SL, Burnham RS, Ravichandiran K, Agur AM, Loh EY. Cadaveric study of sacroiliac joint innervation: Implications for diagnostic blocks and radiofrequency ablation. Reg Anesth Pain Med. 2014;39(6):456–464. doi:10.1097/AAP.0000000000000156. PMID: 25304483.
5. Soto Quijano DA, Otero Loperena E. Sacroiliac joint interventions. Phys Med Rehabil Clin North Am. 2018;29(1):171–183. doi:10.1016/j.pmr.2017.09.004. PMID: 29173661.
6. King W, Ahmed SU, Baisden J, Patel N, Kennedy DJ, Duszynski B, MacVicar J. Diagnosis and treatment of posterior sacroiliac complex pain: A systematic review with comprehensive analysis of the published data. Pain Med. 2015;16(2):257–265. doi:10.1111/pme.12630.
7. Vargas-Salazar M, Venter JA, Finlayson RJ. How I do it: Ultrasound-guided sacral lateral branch blocks. https://www.asra.com/news-publications/asra-newsletter/newsletter-item/asra-news/2020/02/07/how-i-do-it-ultrasound-guided-sacral-lateral-branch-blocks

8. Finlayson RJ, Etheridge JB, Elgueta MF, Thonnagith A, De Villiers F, Nelems B, Tran DQ. A randomized comparison between ultrasound- and fluoroscopy-guided sacral lateral branch blocks. Reg Anesth Pain Med. 2017;42(3):400–406. doi:10.1097/AAP.0000000000000569. PMID: 28178092.
9. Narouze S, Benzon HT, Provenzano D, Buvanendran A, De Andres J, Deer T, Rauck R, Huntoon MA. Interventional spine and pain procedures in patients on antiplatelet and anticoagulant medications (2nd ed.). Reg Anesth Pain Med. 2018;43(3):225–262. doi:10.1097/AAP.0000000000000700. PMID: 29278603.

8

Radiofrequency ablation of the sacroiliac joint

Haider M. Ali, Yashar Eshraghi, and Maged Guirguis

Introduction

Radiofrequency ablation (RFA) is a procedure that results in denervation of the nerves involved in sacroiliac joint (SIJ) pain. It is a treatment that can provide prolonged relief for patients with chronic or refractory SIJ pain.[1-4] RFA is well-established technology that is used not only in pain medicine but also for pathology in other medical specialties such as oncology, cardiology, dermatology, and vascular surgery.[5] In this minimally invasive intervention, probe technology is used percutaneously to create lesions to achieve denervation to the SIJ. It has been shown to be particularly effective for those who have had a positive response to a diagnostic lateral branch block with local anesthetic.[1,2]

Radiofrequency currents are passed through an electrode that is placed near a nociceptive pathway where a predictable lesion is formed (Figure 8.1). The tissue destruction from this lesion is targeted to an area where the responsible nerves traverse.[6] Nerve ablation is a process that leads to death of neurons by way of axonal interruption and nerve fiber degeneration, also known as Wallerian degeneration.[7] This process typically takes time, so patients may not begin to experience relief until several weeks after the procedure.

Although this technique is very effective, its effect is reversible due to nerve regeneration, and pain is expected to recur. For this reason, it is necessary to repeat the procedure to maintain lasting pain relief.[7]

Since the first clinical study regarding RFA procedures to treat SIJ pain in 2001, this procedure has become well established as an effective way to provide significant pain relief for many patients for up to 1 year. The benefits of this treatment approach include prolonged

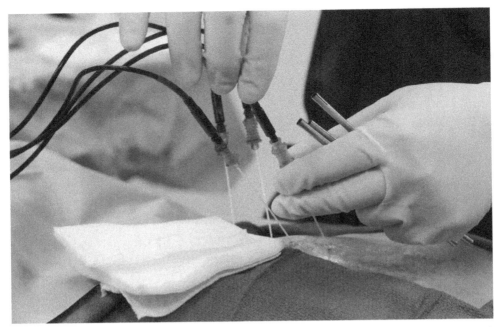

FIGURE 8.1. Electrodes being placed during an RFA procedure. *Source:* PainDoctorUSA, CC BY-SA 4.0 https://creativecommons.org/licenses/by-sa/4.0

pain relief and decreased use of opioids.[4,8] This chapter will present the relevant anatomy, different RFA methods, established evidence from the literature, and clinical outcomes of this treatment approach.

Evidence

In a retrospective study in 2001, Ferrante et al. first described that RFA of the SIJ achieved at least 50% reduction in pain scores in 12 of 33 patients (36.4%), with an average duration of 12 ± 1.2 months.[8] Soon after, in 2003, a retrospective study by Cohen et al. documented at least 50% pain relief in eight of nine patients (88.9%) at 9 months after the procedure. These patients were included based on their successful response to a lateral branch block.[1]

A randomized placebo-controlled study found statistically significant positive clinical outcomes for patients who underwent RFA of the SIJ. These patients had improvements in terms of pain, physical function, disability, and quality of life, particularly at the 3-month mark following their procedure.[9] Based on clinical data from nine studies, a meta-analysis in 2010 concluded that of the patients who received RFA for SIJ pain, 60.1% achieved more than 50% relief at the 3-month mark and 49.9% achieved more than 50% relief after 6 months.[3]

This early evidence provided a promising and revolutionary treatment beyond local anesthetic blocks. More recent evidence, along with new and innovative techniques, will be detailed throughout the chapter.

Anatomy

The initial approaches to areas of nerve denervation were based on creating lesions on the nerves supplying the joint, within the joint itself, or in both locations. Denervation of the posterior joint nerve supply proved to have the most success.[10] The major innervation of the posterior SIJ consists of at least the lateral branches of the L4–S3 dorsal rami.[10,11] A study that compared anatomic differences in RFA techniques for SIJ pain measured capture rates of the sacral lateral branch nerves. The researchers discovered a 100% capture rate at levels S1–S2, 88% at S3, 8% at L5, and 4% at S4.[12] In general, with high anatomic variation of the posterior nerve supply, there is theoretically a higher chance of coverage with the procedure if a larger area is treated.

In contrast, the anterior SIJ is innervated by the posterior rami of L1–S2 as well as by superior gluteal and obturator nerves, which cannot effectively be targeted by RFA.[13]

As previously mentioned, success of the RFA procedure is based on the response to the lateral branch block.[1,2] In the pilot study by Cohen et al. mentioned earlier, the nine patients who were offered the RFA procedure first received L4 and L5 dorsal rami and S1–S3 lateral branch blocks. All these patients were offered RFA, and eight of the nine achieved at least 50% pain relief following the procedure.[1]

The anatomic differences between intraarticular and extraarticular approaches were well detailed by Dreyfuss et al. in a double-blind, randomized, placebo-controlled study. First, it was demonstrated that sacral lateral branches are responsible for pain originating from extraarticular portions of the SIJ. Based on anesthesia to and around the joints, the findings implied that the SIJ has additional innervation beyond the sacral lateral branches, and that lateral branch blocks are particularly useful for identifying pain originating from posterior sacroiliac ligaments. This suggests that lateral branch blocks cannot necessarily be replaced but can be complemented by intraarticular blocks.[14]

Generally, the different anatomic approaches (which involve various methods, described later in the chapter) all involve lesioning to capture the L4–L5 dorsal rami and the lateral branches of S1–S3. The latter are targeted laterally along the dorsal sacral foramina (Figure 8.2).

Based on multiple studies, it has been recommended for electrodes to be placed at least 7 mm from the posterior sacral foramina in order to prevent inadvertent damage to spinal nerves.[11,15]

Co-administration

Prior evidence has shown a positive correlation between size of RFA lesions and content of a preinjected fluid such as sodium chloride, which is known to significantly increase lesion sizes.[16–18] Preinjection with sodium chloride can decrease electrical impedance while increasing thermal conductivity. This combination facilitates electrical delivery and heat transfer, resulting in a larger lesion.[18,19]

Antibiotics are not indicated for this procedure because with appropriate sterile technique, risk for infection is extremely low.

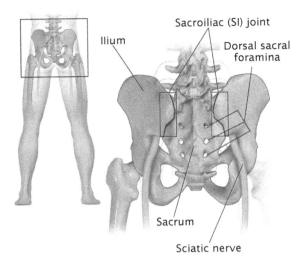

FIGURE 8.2. The sacroiliac joint. *Source:* Blausen.com staff (2014). "Medical gallery of Blausen Medical 2014". WikiJournal of Medicine 1 (2). DOI:10.15347/wjm/2014.010. ISSN 2002-4436, CC BY 3.0 https://creativecommons.org/licenses/by/3.0, modified

Although not routinely practiced, some interventionalists administer steroids along with the procedure to prevent post-neurotomy neuritis. The limited evidence on this practice may bring it into question. One study concluded that injection of steroids before performing RFA reduced the size of the lesion, potentially decreasing chances of success.[19] One study found that the administration of corticosteroids even after RFA did not reduce the incidence of post-neurotomy neuritis.[20]

Methods and procedural technique

The techniques used to achieve denervation have evolved throughout the years, with improved efficiency and varying outcomes. This procedure is done under conscious sedation, with fluoroscopic guidance, and uses needle probes and radiofrequency equipment. The procedure involves secure placement of a dispersive ground pad, measuring electrical impedance, administering nerve stimulation, and monitoring other parameters prior to and during lesioning.

The reason for measuring the electrical impedance is to ensure the circuit is continuous. Ensuring an impedance range of 300 to 700 ohms is helpful in confirming proper electrode placement, in case the electrode may be too close to either vascular tissue or bone. It may also give insight into the integrity of the radiofrequency system, prompting the practitioner to inspect the equipment if the impedances are out of range.

Ground pads or dispersive electrodes are used during RFA to serve as a return path for applied radiofrequency currents. These pads are typically flexible electrical conductors that are coated in an adhesive polymer gel and attached firmly to the patient's skin. The radiofrequency current leaves the body through the large surface area of the pad and thus prevents the temperature from getting to the point of causing an epidermal burn. This risk is further minimized by placing the pad in a location that is ideally as far away from the radiofrequency electrode as possible. This is because the distance between the pad and the electrode is inversely related to the temperature generated.[21] For example, the pad may be placed on the patient's calf opposite to the side of the procedure.

Radiofrequency cannulas with active tips are inserted to the level of the bone. The location of insertion is based on targeting the dorsal rami branches for the SIJ, typically L4–L5 dorsal rami and the lateral branches of S1–S3. Local anesthetic and/or other preinjected fluids can be given via the cannulas prior to electrode placement. Nerve stimulation at 2 Hz with 1 to 3 V of electrical potential is performed to ensure no motor nerves are affected.[7] Sensory stimulation at 50 Hz is also used by some practitioners to guide electrode placement. This may be used in order to account for anatomic variation and to ensure lesions will not be created too close to the dorsal root ganglion.[7]

Once appropriate placement is confirmed and subsequent testing is complete, the practitioner can proceed with creation of the lesions. Other parameters monitored during the procedure include temperature, voltage, current, and wattage. The most widely used methods will be described here, along with their procedural and clinical advantages.

Conventional RFA

The conventional monopolar technique uses thermal probes with temperatures that are typically up to 90°C for up to 120 seconds to create single lesions to disrupt the nerves. Reliable tissue destruction typically begins when the tissue itself reaches a temperature of 60°C.[7] This approach has largely been replaced by upgraded techniques.

Cooled RFA

One of the first successful innovations of RFA came with the introduction of cooled RFA (c-RFA).[22] This technology uses circulating water that is cooled alongside a radiofrequency current to create a monopolar lesion for denervation. By cooling the tip of the needle, this method allows for more consistent energy delivery at the tip, resulting in a larger lesion size. Needle tips are typically maintained around 60°C for several minutes.[12,23] Compared to the conventional method, lesions in c-RFA can be more than double in size and are more likely to denervate nociceptive input from the joint. This larger lesion is more likely to be effective due to the anatomic variation seen in the nerve supply for the SIJ. It is important to note, however, that the larger lesion created with c-RFA does not translate into a longer duration of pain relief.[10]

It has been suggested that the c-RFA method was shown to provide a higher percentage of positive outcomes when compared to the conventional thermal method.[24] Although it is widely accepted as a safe and effective method, this finding was not statistically powered in its claim.[22,25]

Bipolar RFA

The bipolar RFA technique is a more recent and revolutionary method in which two adjacent needle electrodes, with temperatures similar to those used in the conventional method, are positioned in a manner to create a strip lesion.

In a large cadaveric fluoroscopy study by Roberts et al., lesions created by multiple versions of seven current RFA techniques for the SIJ were compared in terms of their efficacy of capturing sacral lateral branch nerves. Overall, a statistically significant finding demonstrated that the bipolar techniques were more successful than the conventional monopolar techniques in terms of percentages of lateral branches captured. There were no statistically significant findings among the different bipolar techniques. The findings in this study also suggested that the current needle placement locations of monopolar techniques may not be able to capture all lateral branches.[12]

Compared to c-RFA, the bipolar method has been deemed less complex by some researchers, with reduced operating time, x-ray exposure, and cost.[26,27]

Some evidence describes further success when distance was increased between the lesions. In 2016, a randomized controlled study found prolonged relief (50% relief at the 12-month mark) with a modified bipolar "palisade" RFA technique where the needle distance was greater than 1 cm, as opposed to exactly 1 cm in the previously described method (<25% relief at the 12-month mark).[28]

A multi-lesion Simplicity probe has also been used in practice. This device offers simultaneous lesioning in a strip with the benefit of a single needle insertion.[29,30] The special probe has three electrodes and can be used to create a continuous and gapless strip lesion, with the option to use just two electrodes to create a smaller lesion.

Pulsed RFA

The techniques described thus far are based on creating lesions with a continuous radiofrequency current. In contrast, another newer method proposed is based on the use of a pulsed current. Uniquely, the pulsed approach does not ablate or create a lesion.[31] It uses less energy and lower temperatures (usually <45°C) to provide "neuromodulation" in a technique that delivers less damage to neurons but still enough to be therapeutic.[5] In theory, this method is intended to be less destructive overall in hopes of reducing post-procedure complications.

Pulsed RFA typically uses a 500-KHz current with a voltage delivery between 45 and 60 V.[5,7] Two bursts are applied per second, with each pulse lasting 20 ms over a 2-minute interval. Due to its mechanism, pulsed RFA should be given for a longer duration and more repeatedly.[7]

The clinical evidence for this technique or its advantages for SIJ pain, however, is limited. Some findings even suggest that pulsed RF is inferior to the earlier-described methods,[32] and there are few studies to support its clinical significance.

A comparative study found that pulsed RF denervation of L4–L5 primary dorsal rami as well as S1–S3 lateral branches provided significant pain relief for patients with SIJ pain.[33] Although optimistic, these findings were based only on comparison to patients who were treated with an intraarticular steroid injection. A literature review of 34 publications yielded promising outcomes specifically for pulsed RF as an effective treatment for sacro-iliac pain as well as for other anatomic locations.[34] The most promising evidence for this technique, specifically for SIJ pain, comes from a clinical trial by Vallejo et al. They found that of patients who underwent pulsed RFA, 72.7% experienced at least 50% reduction in visual analog pain scores.[13]

Summary

In this section, the different RFA methods were presented and compared to provide full historical and clinical context for the interventional proceduralist. With the existing literature, different methods have proven their varying benefits and drawbacks, and therefore most are widely used in practice. Generally, studies have suggested a clinical advantage of the bipolar methods over the rest. This is partly due to the ability to create a strip lesion to account for differences due to anatomic variability. Of note, a systematic review and meta-analysis ranked the effectiveness of the other three RFA techniques from most to least effective at 6-month follow-ups as follows: c-RFA, thermal RFA, and then pulsed RFA.[32] There is certainly a need for continued research to establish the future and direction of RFA techniques.

Drawbacks

The first major limitation to note is the inability of RFA to denervate neurons associated with the anterior SIJ.[2] As described earlier in the chapter, RFA techniques are aimed to target nociceptive input from the posterior SI joint.

Some significant negative associations have been identified as predictors of failures of RFA for SIJ pain. A multivariate analysis found that patients older than 65 who had pain radiating below the knee had a lower chance of success with RFA. In the same study, another negative association was observed with patients who were receiving regular opioid therapy.[24]

Finally, it is important to remember that the pain relief provided by RFA is not permanent.[2] Nerves are expected to regenerate sometime between several months to a year, and this partially accounts for the variability seen in clinical outcomes. The RFA procedure can be repeated to provide sustained relief for patients with significant chronic pain syndromes.

Complications

As with many different types of procedures, there are risks with RFA, including bleeding, burns, infection, nerve damage, and neuritis. The practitioner should take careful steps to prevent unwanted tissue destruction or sensory/motor impairment.

To prevent burns, proper use of the dispersive ground pad (described in detail earlier in the chapter) is mandatory. Aside from maximizing the distance of the pad from the electrodes, the pad can be placed such that the longest side faces the radiofrequency needle to further decrease the risk of a burn.[21] The practitioner should also inspect the radiofrequency cannula for any insulation defects.

Listening to the patient for any complaints of burning or pain during the procedure can alert the practitioner to potential complications. For this reason, a patient who is sedated may be at a higher risk for certain complications.[21]

Special care should be taken for patients with pacemakers or implantable cardioverter–defibrillators (ICDs), as it possible for RFA devices to interfere with their function. Overall, this is not a contraindication and these procedures can be safely performed in these patients. It is recommended, however, to consult a cardiologist or electrophysiologist prior to performing an RFA procedure in this population.[35] There are no reports of RFA procedures causing dysfunction of ICDs or pacemakers in a way that has led to serious injury or death, but there are some steps that can be taken as a precaution. One would be to have a manufacturer's representative present for support in interrogation during the procedure, if needed. Another would be to use a magnet to disable certain devices while using an external defibrillator should arrhythmias occur during a procedure.[35]

Conclusion

RFA is a very effective, modern, and minimally invasive intervention for patients with chronic or refractory SIJ pain. This procedure should be especially considered for patients who have had significant pain relief with a lateral branch block, as the evidence suggests a strong association with positive outcomes.[1,2]

Although there is strong clinical research for SIJ RFA in general, with some data favoring the bipolar methods, most of the methods mentioned in this chapter are still widely used. Some researchers have strongly suggested that there is room for improvement in education for the interventional pain community regarding RFA.[36]

It is evident that more research and clinical trials are necessary to further establish the future of this revolutionary treatment. As we progress through modern medicine, we expect that more innovative devices and techniques will be introduced to the world of interventional pain management. With that said, the exceptional practitioner is one who is well read and up to date on literature and has a patient-centered approach when working to provide the best possible clinical outcomes.

References

1. Cohen SP, Abdi S. Lateral branch blocks as a treatment for sacroiliac joint pain: A pilot study. Reg Anesth Pain Med. 2003;28(2):113–119. doi:10.1053/rapm.2003.50029. PMID: 12677621.
2. Schmidt GL, Bhandutia AK, Altman DT. Management of sacroiliac joint pain. J Am Acad Orthop Surg. 2018;26(17):610–616. doi:10.5435/JAAOS-D-15-00063. PMID: 30059395.
3. Aydin SM, Gharibo CG, Mehnert M, Stitik TP. The role of radiofrequency ablation for sacroiliac joint pain: A meta-analysis. PM R. 2010;2(9):842–851. doi:10.1016/j.pmrj.2010.03.035. PMID: 20869684.
4. Salman O, Gad G, Mohamed AA, Farae HH, Abdelfatah AM. Randomized, controlled blind study comparing sacroiliac intra-articular steroid injection to radiofrequency denervation for sacroiliac joint pain. Egypt J Anaesth. 2015;32(2):219–225. doi:10.1016/j.egja.2015.07.005

5. Cosman ER Jr, Cosman ER Sr. Electric and thermal field effects in tissue around radiofrequency electrodes. Pain Med. 2005;6(6):405–424. doi:10.1111/j.1526-4637.2005.00076.x. PMID: 16336478.
6. Wray JK, Dixon B, Przkora R. Radiofrequency ablation. StatPearls, 2020. https://www.ncbi.nlm.nih.gov/books/NBK482387/
7. Choi EJ, Choi YM, Jang EJ, Kim JY, Kim TK, Kim KH. Neural ablation and regeneration in pain practice. Korean J Pain. 2016;29(1):3–11. doi:10.3344/kjp.2016.29.1.3. PMID: 26839664; PMCID: PMC4731549.
8. Ferrante FM, King LF, Roche EA, Kim PS, Aranda M, Delaney LR, Mardini IA, Mannes AJ. Radiofrequency sacroiliac joint denervation for sacroiliac syndrome. Reg Anesth Pain Med. 2001;26(2):137–142. doi:10.1053/rapm.2001.21739. PMID: 11251137.
9. Patel N, Gross A, Brown L, Gekht G. A randomized, placebo-controlled study to assess the efficacy of lateral branch neurotomy for chronic sacroiliac joint pain. Pain Med. 2012;13(3):383–398. doi:10.1111/j.1526-4637.2012.01328.x. PMID: 22299761.
10. Cohen SP, Hurley RW, Buckenmaier CC 3rd, Kurihara C, Morlando B, Dragovich A. Randomized placebo-controlled study evaluating lateral branch radiofrequency denervation for sacroiliac joint pain. Anesthesiology. 2008;109(2):279–288. doi:10.1097/ALN.0b013e31817f4c7c. PMID: 18648237; PMCID: PMC2666931.
11. Cohen SP. Sacroiliac joint pain: A comprehensive review of anatomy, diagnosis, and treatment. Anesth Analg. 2005;101(5):1440–1453. doi:10.1213/01.ANE.0000180831.60169.EA. PMID: 16244008.
12. Roberts SL, Stout A, Loh EY, Swain N, Dreyfuss P, Agur AM. Anatomical comparison of radiofrequency ablation techniques for sacroiliac joint pain. Pain Med. 2018;19(10):1924–1943. doi:10.1093/pm/pnx329. PMID: 29415262.
13. Vallejo R, Benyamin RM, Kramer J, Stanton G, Joseph NJ. Pulsed radiofrequency denervation for the treatment of sacroiliac joint syndrome. Pain Med. 2006;7(5):429–434. doi:10.1111/j.1526-4637.2006.00143.x. PMID: 17014602.
14. Dreyfuss P, Henning T, Malladi N, Goldstein B, Bogduk N. The ability of multi-site, multi-depth sacral lateral branch blocks to anesthetize the sacroiliac joint complex. Pain Med. 2009;10(4):679–688. doi:10.1111/j.1526-4637.2009.00631.x. PMID: 19638143.
15. Wright RE, Allan KJ, Bainbridge JS. In and ex vivo validation of a novel technique for radiofrequency denervation of the dorsal sacroiliac joint—including a case study. Reg Anesth Pain Med. 2013;38(suppl 1):E161–E162.
16. Provenzano DA, Lassila HC, Somers D. The effect of fluid injection on lesion size during radiofrequency treatment. Reg Anesth Pain Med. 2010;35(4):338–342. doi:10.1097/aap.0b013e3181e82d44. PMID: 20607874.
17. Provenzano DA, Liebert MA, Somers DL. Increasing the NaCl concentration of the preinjected solution enhances monopolar radiofrequency lesion size. Reg Anesth Pain Med. 2013;38(2):112–123. doi:10.1097/AAP.0b013e31827d18f3. PMID: 23388614.
18. Goldberg SN, Ahmed M, Gazelle GS, Kruskal JB, Huertas JC, Halpern EF, Oliver BS, Lenkinski RE. Radio-frequency thermal ablation with NaCl solution injection: Effect of electrical conductivity on tissue heating and coagulation-phantom and porcine liver study. Radiology. 2001;219(1):157–165. doi:10.1148/radiology.219.1.r01ap27157. PMID: 11274551.
19. Tiyaprasertkul W, Perez J. Injection of steroids before radiofrequency ablation has a negative impact on lesion size. Reg Anesth Pain Med. 2014;39(3):189–191. doi:10.1097/AAP.0000000000000067. PMID: 24646623.
20. Singh JR, Miccio VF Jr, Modi DJ, Sein MT. The impact of local steroid administration on the incidence of neuritis following lumbar facet radiofrequency neurotomy. Pain Physician. 2019;22(1):69–74. PMID: 30700070.
21. McCormick ZL, Smith CC, Engel AJ; Spine Intervention Society's Patient Safety Committee. Preventing external skin burns during thermal radiofrequency neurotomy. Pain Med. 2019;20(4):852–853. doi:10.1093/pm/pny274. PMID: 30590703.
22. Karaman H, Kavak GO, Tüfek A, Çelik F, Yildirim ZB, Akdemir MS, Tokgöz O. Cooled radiofrequency application for treatment of sacroiliac joint pain. Acta Neurochir. 2011;153(7):1461–1468. doi:10.1007/s00701-011-1003-8. PMID: 21479801.

23. Kapural L, Deering JP. A technological overview of cooled radiofrequency ablation and its effectiveness in the management of chronic knee pain. Pain Manag. 2020;10(3):133–140. doi:10.2217/pmt-2019-0066. PMID: 32167418.

24. Cohen SP, Strassels SA, Kurihara C, Crooks MT, Erdek MA, Forsythe A, Marcuson M. Outcome predictors for sacroiliac joint (lateral branch) radiofrequency denervation. Reg Anesth Pain Med. 2009;34(3):206–214. doi:10.1097/AAP.0b013e3181958f4b. PMID: 19587617.

25. Cosman ER Jr, Gonzalez CD. Bipolar radiofrequency lesion geometry: Implications for palisade treatment of sacroiliac joint pain. Pain Pract. 2011;11(1):3–22. doi:10.1111/j.1533-2500.2010.00400.x. PMID: 20602716.

26. Burnham RS, Yasui Y. An alternate method of radiofrequency neurotomy of the sacroiliac joint: A pilot study of the effect on pain, function, and satisfaction. Reg Anesth Pain Med. 2007;32(1):12–19. doi:10.1016/j.rapm.2006.08.008. PMID: 17196487.

27. Cheng J, Chen SL, Zimmerman N, Dalton JE, LaSalle G, Rosenquist R. A new radiofrequency ablation procedure to treat sacroiliac joint pain. Pain Physician. 2016;19(8):603–615. PMID: 27906939.

28. Cánovas Martínez L, Orduña VJ, Paramés ME, Lamelas RL, Rojas GS, Domínguez GM. Sacroiliac joint pain: Prospective, randomised, experimental and comparative study of thermal radiofrequency with sacroiliac joint block. Rev Esp Anestesiol Reanim. 2016;63(5):267–272. doi:10.1016/j.redar.2015.08.003

29. Bayerl SH, Finger T, Heiden P, Esfahani-Bayerl N, Topar C, Prinz V, Woitzik J, Dengler J, Vajkoczy P. Radiofrequency denervation for treatment of sacroiliac joint pain: Comparison of two different ablation techniques. Neurosurg Rev. 2020;43(1):101–107. doi:10.1007/s10143-018-1016-3. PMID: 30066034.

30. Schmidt PC, Pino CA, Vorenkamp KE. Sacroiliac joint radiofrequency ablation with a multilesion probe: A case series of 60 patients. Anesth Analg. 2014;119(2):460–462. doi:10.1213/ANE.0000000000000282. PMID: 25046790.

31. Byrd D, Mackey S. Pulsed radiofrequency for chronic pain. Curr Pain Headache Rep. 2008;12(1):37–41. doi: 10.1007/s11916-008-0008-3. PMID: 18417022; PMCID: PMC2913603.

32. Shih CL, Shen PC, Lu CC, Liu ZM, Tien YC, Huang PJ, Chou SH. A comparison of efficacy among different radiofrequency ablation techniques for the treatment of lumbar facet joint and sacroiliac joint pain: A systematic review and meta-analysis. Clin Neurol Neurosurg. 2020;195:105854. doi:10.1016/j.clineuro.2020.105854. PMID: 32353665.

33. Dutta K, Dey S, Bhattacharyya P, Agarwal S, Dev P. Comparison of efficacy of lateral branch pulsed radiofrequency denervation and intraarticular depot methylprednisolone injection for sacroiliac joint pain. Pain Physician. 2018;21(5):489–496. PMID: 30282393.

34. Boudier-Revéret M, Thu AC, Hsiao MY, Shyu SG, Chang MC. The effectiveness of pulsed radiofrequency on joint pain: A narrative review. Pain Pract. 2020;20(4):412–421. doi:10.1111/papr.12863. PMID: 31782970.

35. Smith C, DeFrancesch F, Patel J; Spine Intervention Society's Patient Safety Committee. Radiofrequency neurotomy for facet joint pain in patients with permanent pacemakers and defibrillators. Pain Med. 2019;20(2):411–412. doi:10.1093/pm/pny213. PMID: 30358865.

36. Provenzano DA, Buvanendran A, de León-Casasola OA, Narouze S, Cohen SP. Interpreting the MINT randomized trials evaluating radiofrequency ablation for lumbar facet and sacroiliac joint pain: A call from ASRA for better education, study design, and performance. Reg Anesth Pain Med. 2018;43(1):68–71. doi:10.1097/AAP.0000000000000699

PART III

Role of regenerative medicine

9

Regenerative medicine therapies for sacroiliac joint disease

Natalie H. Strand, Jillian Maloney, and Christine L. Hunt

Introduction

The sacroiliac joint (SIJ) is a common cause of chronic pain, responsible for up to 30% of patients with chronic low back pain.[1,2] Common treatments for SIJ-related pain include physical therapy, pharmacologic treatments, and interventional treatments. Interventional treatments include intraarticular steroid injections and lateral branch radiofrequency ablation (RFA). As interest from both patients and physicians increases in the field of regenerative medicine, a thorough understanding of biologic-based interventional techniques, including prolotherapy, stem cell therapy, platelet-rich plasma (PRP), autologous whole blood, and hyaluronic acid, for the treatment of SIJ-related pain is mandatory. In this chapter we will review the various regenerative injectants available, their mechanisms of action, efficacy, possible adverse effects, and formulations and will provide a brief review of clinical trials and published data.

Prolotherapy

Background

The principle of promoting healing via injection of an irritant has been present since the time of Hippocrates. However, modern prolotherapy,[3] also known as regenerative injection therapy, was first described in 1937.[4] The National Institutes of Health categorizes prolotherapy as complementary and alternative medicine.[5] The basic concept is that the injection of an irritating substance into a painful site will promote healing and strengthen ligaments, leading to reduced pain.[5] Prolotherapy was initially used to treat pain in the setting

TABLE 9.1 Injectants for prolotherapy

Type of injectant	Example	Mechanism of action
Osmotic agent	Hyperosmolar dextrose, zinc sulfate, glycerin	Dehydration/"osmotic shock"
Irritant	Phenol, guaiacol, pumic acid	Damage to cell membranes
Chemotactic agent	Sodium morrhuate	Direct chemotactic agent to inflammatory cells

of ligamentous laxity with the aim of reducing hypermobility but has since been expanded to multiple other areas, to include axial joints. According to the *Journal of Prolotherapy*'s consensus statement on prolotherapy, physical exam findings that point to usefulness of prolotherapy include laxity of a joint and tender points where tendons or ligaments attach to bones. Conditions that may benefit include degenerative osteoarthritis and ligamentous laxity. Prolotherapy injections to treat SIJ-related pain can be intraarticular or periarticular to target sacral ligamentous laxity.[6]

Injectants are widely classified into three subgroups (Table 9.1): osmotic agents, irritants, and chemotactic agents. Hypertonic dextrose is thought to act by osmotic shock, or rupture of cells.[5] Phenol is believed to cause cellular irritation and damage cell membranes. Morrhuate sodium is believed to be a direct chemotactic agent and results in local release of inflammatory mediators.[7]

Pharmacology

The exact mechanism of action of prolotherapy is not known,[5] but it is widely accepted that the basic premise is that prolotherapy promotes healing by initiating an acute inflammatory response. There are several theories as to why this therapy may promote healing. Injection of an irritating solution is thought to induce localized inflammation. Ultimately, fibroblasts congregate and are thought to result in deposition of collagen in the area.[7] Prolotherapy may help with sacroiliac pain related to joint hypermobility or excess laxity by promoting ligament repair and reducing clinical instability. Growth factors may be stimulated by prolotherapy and may contribute to tissue response.[12] These hypotheses are not unrefuted, and a rat model has shown that the inflammatory response from prolotherapy injections was not different from needle trauma alone.[13]

Intraarticular prolotherapy may provide improvement to the ventral structures of the SIJ. Given that ventral pathology has been shown to be present in up to 69% of patients with positive responses to SIJ diagnostic blocks,[14] the potential for intraarticular prolotherapy to target these ventral structures may be an important differentiator as these are inaccessible to RFA denervation of the SIJ.

Studies have shown that the effects of SIJ prolotherapy can last up to and beyond 2 years.[15] While many protocols recommend three to six (or more) series of injections spaced 2 to 6 weeks apart, some data support that patients who do not respond at all after the first injection are unlikely to experience meaningful pain improvement or functional gains overall.[16]

Data on safety and efficacy

Yelland et al. reviewed randomized and quasi-randomized controlled trials (RCTs) that compared prolotherapy injections to control injections for chronic low back pain.[17] While not specific for SIJ pain, they did identify that evidence was conflicting with regard to prolotherapy injections helping with disability related to low back pain. There were no data to support that prolotherapy injections used in isolation were more successful than control injections. Interestingly, when combined with co-therapies, prolotherapy injections were deemed more efficacious than control injections.

Rabago et al. performed a systematic review of prolotherapy for chronic musculoskeletal pain.[18] They identified 34 case reports and case series and six RCTs. The data were conflicting, and they ultimately concluded that existing studies are "far from definitive" and that while prolotherapy appears safe, it is unclear who may benefit the most from prolotherapy for musculoskeletal pain.

Animal studies have shown that 5% sodium morrhuate sclerosing injection strengthened patellar tendons in rats.[19] Human studies have demonstrated improved ligament stability in the anterior cruciate ligament after hyperosmolar dextrose injections.[20]

One prospective RCT evaluated the efficacy of intraarticular SIJ prolotherapy (25% dextrose, two or three injections at 2-week intervals) to improve SIJ pain compared to intraarticular steroid injections in the same location and found that while the pain and disability scores were improved in both groups, the percentage of patients with greater than 50% pain improvement at 15 months was 58% in the prolotherapy group and only 10% in the steroid group.[21] The conclusion was that intraarticular prolotherapy with 5% dextrose in water could be beneficial for the treatment of SIJ pain in the long term.

Cusi et al. performed a prospective descriptive study to evaluate the effectiveness of three injections of hypertonic dextrose (18% dextrose) into the dorsal interosseous ligament of the affected SIJ under computed tomography (CT) guidance at 6-week intervals for three series. They determined that the patients in the study confirmed the hypothesis that the injections would increase the stiffness of the dorsal interosseous ligament.[15] They showed an improvement in the Quebec Back Pain Disability Scale of 20 points 3 months after treatment, and the improvement in disability remained significant up to 2 years later.

Hoffman and Agnish examined the effectiveness of SIJ prolotherapy for SIJ instability with a retrospective cohort study reviewing the experiences of 103 patients with low back pain and SIJ instability.[16] Each patient underwent three intraarticular SIJ prolotherapy injections spaced 4 weeks apart with 15% dextrose in lidocaine (7 mL 1% lidocaine and 3 mL 50% dextrose). Functional gains were measured with the Oswestry Disability Index, and 23% showed an improvement of 15 points at follow-up, approximately 50% showed no improvement, and 29% had improvement of less than 15 points. Interestingly, patients who did not improve after the initial injection were not likely to improve after three injections.

Overall, additional trials are needed to examine and validate the use of prolotherapy for SIJ pain. The optimal concentrations, volumes, time intervals, total number of injections, and formulations are yet to be determined. The predominant risks of prolotherapy are related to the injection itself, with needle trauma having the potential to cause bleeding, bruising, swelling, and infection. There is a risk of allergic and anaphylactic responses to injected agents.[11] One review concluded that minor side effects were common but transient and included back pain and stiffness.[17]

Preparation and administration

Several injectants have been used in the past,[8] but the most common is hypertonic dextrose.[9] Hypertonic dextrose is thought to initiate regeneration of damaged intraarticular tissue, including cartilage and ligaments, and is categorized as regenerative injection therapy.[10] The inflammatory concentration of hypertonic dextrose is typically 12.5% to 25%. The recommended interval between injections is 4 to 6 weeks, with the average person requiring three to six treatments in total.[11]

Mesenchymal stem cells

Background

In his reflections on the morphology of lymph tissue and the appearance of unique cells for which he argued the term "stem cell" seemed most appropriate, Dr. Edward Gall contributed to the earliest discussion regarding the definition of the lineage of stem cells and their multipotent potential.[22] Just as electron microscopy revolutionized the pathologist's understanding of cellular structure and provided insight leading to the discovery of the function of mesenchymal stem cells (MSCs), so have advances in flow cytometry and molecular characterization techniques shifted the focus on use of MSCs from pioneering scientific development to a field that is increasingly scrutinized, with an emphasis on understanding the mechanisms of this therapy and its appropriate clinical applications. MSCs have been studied in many different types of research and clinical applications, including cardiac, neurologic, hepatobiliary, endocrine, renal, autoimmune, lung, and periodontal disease.[23] MSCs can be harvested from several sources in human tissue, but in point-of-care musculoskeletal pain applications including SIJ pain, the most common sources are bone marrow and adipose. Due to current U.S. Food and Drug Administration (FDA) guidance, the most feasible source for MSC harvest is bone marrow, and thus the rest of this section will focus on bone marrow–derived MSCs (B-MSCs). Adipose-derived MSCs may be prepared using enzymatic degradation or mechanical centrifugation.

Dating back to their original characterization as colony-forming units-fibroblastic (CFU-F) due to their fibroblast-like appearance and ability to adhere to plastic, MSCs are historically defined as cells able to adhere to plastic in standard culture, must express specific cell surface markers (CD105[+], CD73[+], CD90[+], CD45[-], CD34[-], CD14[-] or CD11b[-], CD79alpha[-], CD19[-], HLA-DR[-]), and must possess trilineage potential with the ability to differentiate into osteoblasts, adipocytes, or chondroblasts in vitro.[24] Considerable discussion regarding a more specific phenotype to define MSCs has arisen since the original consensus statement in 2006. It is likely that the antibody Stro-1 may be a key component of the in vivo MSC phenotype.

Pharmacology

The study of MSCs in vivo has revealed that transplanted MSCs in musculoskeletal application do not engraft or indeed persist beyond 2 weeks or so in most conditions. The mechanism of action of MSCs is thought to lie in their trophic and paracrine as well as immunomodulatory effects. MSC transplantation results in cell-to-cell communication and paracrine secretion of bioactive molecules that may aid in repair of musculoskeletal tissue and help direct differentiation of endogenous progenitor cells into osteoblasts and chondroblasts. The trophic effects of MSCs are thought to be due to secreted factors including growth factors, morphogens, chemokines, cytokines, exosomes or extracellular vesicles, and glycosaminoglycans.[25] Collectively these molecules help direct the local microenvironment toward an anti-inflammatory, pro-reparative milieu for musculoskeletal tissue. The characterization of extracellular vesicles and the significance of their role in musculoskeletal tissue repair is an important area of ongoing research in the field of regenerative medicine.[26]

The immunomodulatory effects of MSCs are thought to lie in the secretion of molecules that interact with immune cells to modulate the activity of immune cells including B cells, T cells, natural killer cells, and dendritic cells.[25] These cytokines and molecules include nitric oxide, prostaglandin E2 (PGE2), indoleamine 2, 3-dioxygenase (IDO), interleukin-10 (IL-10), and transforming growth factor-beta 1 (TGFβ1) and are thought to interact with immune cells, resulting in anti-inflammatory and regenerative effects. As our understanding of the role of MSCs has evolved, interest lies in their likely origin as perivascular cells. Although their characterization as true "pericytes" is controversial, MSCs likely represent adventitial cells that act as precursors to multiple cell types, including pericytes. This would explain their predilection toward being activated during tissue injury, shifting from their role as progenitor cells residing in the adventitial layer of blood cells during homeostasis to an activated state directed toward engagement in tissue repair at the site of local injury.[27,28]

The isolation, characterization, and optimization of the trophic, paracrine, and immunomodulatory effects of MSCs remain dynamic areas of research.[29] Cultured MSCs from bone marrow, adipose, and other tissue sources can be genetically modified or lineage directed to favor specific progenitor cell lines and possibly directed toward specific treatment of disease or injury. The current regulatory environment precludes more than minimal manipulation of harvested tissue, and thus these areas of research remain important areas to monitor to improve our understanding of the safety and effectiveness of MSC therapies in the treatment of musculoskeletal disease, including SIJ pain.

The concept of MSCs as "medicine" has led to Dr. Arnold Caplan's proposal that these cells are more aptly described as "medicinal signaling cells."[30,31] MSCs likely function to recruit endogenous pericytes to local tissue where they are injected, with the observed resultant effects of tissue repair, inflammation reduction, and pain improvement lying in the body's own endogenous response to signal the need for tissue repair persisting far beyond the period of time that engrafted cells remain viable in vivo.

Data on safety and efficacy

Intraarticular SIJ MSC injection may be considered in appropriate candidates with clinical signs and symptoms of SIJ-mediated pain. However, there is a paucity of literature with respect to the safety and efficacy of MSC therapy in SIJ pain specifically. No studies to date have been performed investigating intraarticular SIJ injection of MSCs; however, multiple studies investigating the safety of biologic injections in peripheral joints may be considered when evaluating the likely safety in SIJ injections. There have not been any serious adverse effects reported from SIJ injection of MSCs.

No studies to date have been performed investigating intraarticular SIJ injection of MSCs. Regarding evidence for efficacy of MSC therapy for axial low back pain more broadly, there is level I/IV evidence supporting the intradiscal injection of MSCs,[32] with at least three studies[33,34] demonstrating improvement in pain and function through at least 1 year following intradiscal injection and at least one study showing no improvement in pain.[35] The SIJ, however, is more akin to peripheral joints lined with articular cartilage than to the intervertebral disc, and it is reasonable to look to studies performed at other applications to consider the potential effectiveness of injection to the SIJ lined by articular cartilage.

Several RCTs of low to moderate quality have demonstrated improvement in pain and function following B-MSC injection, but all are limited by a high degree of bias and a small study size.[36] A recent meta-analysis of 17 studies investigating the efficacy of MSCs in the treatment of pain and loss of function due to knee osteoarthritis included six RCTs, three prospective observational studies, and three retrospective case-control studies. Fifteen of the 17 studies reported improvement in clinical outcomes, nine of 11 studies reported improvement of cartilage status on magnetic resonance imaging (MRI), and six of seven studies reported evidence of tissue repair on arthroscopy.[37] All studies involving autologous MSCs and all observational and case-control studies were determined to have a high risk of bias. Only one study was considered to be of high quality according to Grading of Recommendations, Assessment, Development, and Evaluation (GRADE) guidelines. Overall the authors were unable to make firm determinations with respect to the efficacy of MSCs in terms of clinical outcomes for knee osteoarthritis including pain, function, and cartilage repair due to the heterogeneity of cell preparation and methods of administration, quality of the evidence, and use of adjuvant treatments to varying degrees.

There is clearly a paucity of evidence with respect to the safety and efficacy of intraarticular MSC injections for SIJ-mediated pain. Although studies investigating potential effects of MSCs on cartilaginous joints are promising, there is no consensus based on high-quality studies regarding the effectiveness of MSCs for intraarticular joint pain and disability or cartilage repair.

Preparation and administration

Ultimately, the efficacy of MSCs in musculoskeletal applications may depend on the ability to select for appropriately homogenous MSCs based on cell surface receptor antigen expression in cultured colonies, but MSCs currently available for use in point-of-care clinical practice may not undergo more than minimal manipulation. Enzymatic degradation is considered by the FDA to involve more than minimal manipulation and thus cannot be performed outside of a research context, and mechanical centrifugation of harvested adipose requires a specific method of preparation that may not be accessible in some clinical settings.[38] Thus, the method for harvesting and preparation of B-MSCs is described here.

The FDA has issued several guidance memos regulating the use of human cells, tissues, and cellular and tissue-based products (HCT/Ps). Unless HCT/Ps meet specific criteria, they require FDA-regulated study under an Investigational New Drug (IND) application and premarket approval before they can be made available for commercial use. Such products are regulated as a drug or biologic. HCT/Ps meeting the following criteria are currently considered exempt from FDA regulation under Section 351 of the Public Health Service Act:

1. Products undergoing minimal manipulation
2. Products intended for homologous use
3. The preparation of HCT/P does not involve combination with another agent other than water, crystalloids, or a sterilizing, preservative, or storage agent
4. The product is intended for autologous use (or first- or second-degree relative allogeneic transplantation) if they are expected to have a systemic effect. [39]

HCT/Ps meeting these criteria are regulated instead under Section 361 of the Public Health Service Act and 21 CFR 1271. For structural tissue including bone, blood vessel, or adipose, "minimal manipulation" means that processing does not alter the relevant characteristics of the tissue related to its utility for reconstruction, repair, or replacement. "Homologous use" is defined as the product performs the same basic function in the donor and recipient tissue (which has historically been taken to mean taken from one site within the same host and applied to another). The FDA defines "basic" function as that which is apparent from a biologic or physiologic point of view. The FDA has explicitly stated that the use of HCT/Ps from adipose for the treatment of a degenerative or inflammatory disorder is generally considered to be non-homologous use, specifically including arthritis or tendinitis. PRP is considered to be outside the scope of this guidance as it is not considered to be HCT/Ps. The FDA has stated that minimally manipulated bone marrow intended for homologous use that has not undergone more than minimal manipulation and not combined with another article (except as noted earlier) is also not considered HCT/P. Thus, both the method of preparation and the intended use of B-MSCs is critical for considering whether a product requires FDA regulation under Section 361 or can be considered exempt from such regulation. The FDA regularly updates this guidance, and pain practitioners should ensure they remain up to date with the latest regulatory guidance and regulatory framework. This summarizes the latest FDA guidance regarding regulation of MSCs and HCT/Ps, but the regulatory environment continues to evolve as the field of regenerative medicine expands and the FDA makes continuous efforts to appropriately regulate this rapidly expanding area of research and clinical practice.

Hernigou et al. describe the key anatomic structures and safety considerations with bone marrow harvest using a trocar needle as is typically performed in regenerative medicine procedures harvesting B-MSCs.[40] Risk of violation of or injury to key vascular or neurologic structures is higher in obese patients and with less experienced practitioners. Key structures to consider for safety with bone marrow aspirate harvest include the sciatic nerve and superior gluteal vessel and the external iliac artery. Although the risk of bone marrow aspiration is lower than bone graft harvesting in terms of complications, there is risk of injury to neurologic structures and blood vessels, potentially leading to neurologic injury, hematoma, and even injury to soft tissue structures that may require operative repair. Therefore, some form of image assistance is recommended, as is appropriate training with an experienced practitioner. There is no universally accepted approach to the bone marrow aspiration, although thanks in large part to the work of Hernigou, a posterior approach is often used.

Herein we describe the method of preparation and administration of intraarticular SIJ injection using B-MSCs that meet the criteria mentioned earlier of minimal manipulation, homologous use, autologous delivery, and not in combination with another drug or biologic according to the current understanding of regulatory guidance. Bone marrow currently is typically harvested from the posterior iliac crest, with the patient in the supine position. Harvest of bone marrow is generally conducted with ultrasound assistance or fluoroscopic guidance. The ultrasound-assisted procedure typically involves placement of the ultrasound probe over the posterior superior iliac spine (PSIS), taking care to ensure the target is appropriately visualized. The patient is sterilely prepped and draped and aseptic technique is used throughout. The superficial tissues are anesthetized using local anesthetic, and a 1-cm stab incision is made over the PSIS. Shapiro et al. describe their recommended trajectory of the bone marrow aspiration needle and aspirate yield per position, not advancing further than 4 cm into the bone of the ilium from the PSIS to avoid the risk of penetrating the lateral or medial edges of the iliac crest.[41] They describe using a total of four advancements or "passes" into the iliac crest, with aspiration of 5 to 8 mL at each location.

Bone marrow aspiration can also be conducted with CT or fluoroscopic guidance. A retrospective imaging study of 260 patients using 3D reconstructed CT images demonstrated that a needle trajectory approach from the PSIS to the anterior inferior iliac spine (AIIS) allowed for a safe approach staying greater than 1 cm above the greater sciatic notch in all subjects, within a large area of cancellous bone for higher-quality marrow harvest.[42] Figure 9.1 shows this approach. In this proposed fluoroscopically guided technique, the PSIS and AIIS are superimposed radiographically in a "teardrop merging view," with the bone marrow aspirate trocar advanced coaxially from the PSIS to the AIIS to a maximum depth of 6 cm. Figure 9.2 shows an example of this. Aspirate yields of 3 to 5 mL of bone marrow are withdrawn at 6 cm of depth, the needle is rotated 90 degrees and withdrawn slightly, and the procedure is repeated for a maximum of 30 mL of aspirate with a single passage of the trocar through the iliac crest. This technique may allow for safe and high-quality aspiration of bone marrow with minimal patient morbidity. Regardless of aspiration technique, further study is needed to validate CFU-F per mL with various approaches and large-N studies to examine the safety of bone marrow aspiration techniques for regenerative medicine applications. As described earlier, point-of-care MSC preparation must be performed using minimal manipulation and not combined with any other drug or biologic

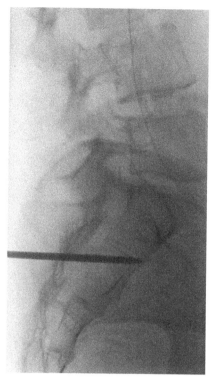

FIGURE 9.1. Lateral view of the proposed fluoroscopically guided bone marrow aspiration approach. GSN = greater sciatic notch; S1 = S1 vertebral body.

agent when administered. A variety of centrifuges are commercially available. The processing method can vary widely depending on the device used, but it is recommended to only use devices authorized by the FDA for centrifugation of bone marrow aspirate in preparation of B-MSCs using only the appropriate vendor-recommended anticoagulant for point-of-care preparation. Unlike PRP, there is no universally accepted definition for the appropriate concentrate of bone marrow aspirate; however, most devices will allow the practitioner to specify a hematocrit setting to produce leukocyte-rich or leukocyte-poor product, depending on the intended use. The operator and all assistants should undergo appropriate training and follow standard operating procedures for aspiration and preparation of B-MSCs.

After the bone marrow has been concentrated in the centrifuge, the product is ready for injection. The SIJ can be appropriately visualized under fluoroscopy or ultrasound according to standard procedure, and contrast or gadolinium is injected to confirm intraarticular spread pattern if using fluoroscopy. Bone marrow aspirate concentrate is then injected, using a recommended standard volume of not more than 3 mL to avoid over-pressurizing the joint. The needle is then withdrawn. It is not recommended to use local anesthetic in the joint or with withdrawal of the needle due to the chondrotoxicity of lidocaine to human MSCs.[43]

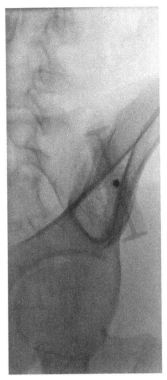

FIGURE 9.2. "Teardrop-merging" view of the proposed fluoroscopically guided bone marrow aspiration approach. The posterior superior iliac spine (PSIS) and anterior inferior iliac spine (AIIS) are radiographically superimposed, and the trocar is directed along the upper portion of the teardrop to remain above the greater sciatic notch and within the walls of the ilium. IL = Ilium; A/P = superimposed PSIS and AIIS; asterisk = trocar needle in coaxial view.

Platelet-Rich Plasma

Background

PRP is derived from autologous blood. The main component of PRP is platelets, with platelet levels significantly greater than the baseline count in whole blood. PRP has been used since the 1980s in surgical practices but has recently gained popularity and interest in treating musculoskeletal injuries such as tendon and ligament injuries,[44–46] knee osteoarthritis,[47,48] and muscle strains.[44] Platelets contain proteins, cytokines, and other factors that participate in wound healing.[49] The aim of PRP is to administer a high concentration of platelet growth factors to injured tissue to promote healing.[49]

Pharmacology

There are several theories on the regenerative mechanism of action of PRP. It is thought to be mediated by growth factors such as platelet-derived growth factor (PDGF) subunits A, B, and C; transforming growth factor beta1 (TGF-Beta1); insulin-like growth factor 1 (IGF-1); fibroblast growth factor 3 (FGF-2); hepatocyte growth factor (HGF); and vascular endothelial growth factor A (VEGF-A), which enhance tissue recovery.[47] VEGF and FGF2 stimulate angiogenesis.[47] PRP causes secretion of chemokines, which signals leukocytes to infiltrate the damaged tissue, thus initiating the inflammatory response.[47] Platelets also secrete cell adhesion molecules like fibrinogen and fibronectin; this is thought to help cell migration.[49]

After platelet activation, about 70% of growth factors are secreted within 10 minutes, with the nearly 30% remaining secreted within an hour.[50] How this translates clinically into onset of action, however, is unclear and depends on many variables, including platelet concentration of the PRP, preparation of injectate, volume injected, and location injected. The ideal dose for SIJ injections has not been determined. A series of injections can be administered, and the determination is based on responsiveness, degree of pathology, and provider experience. Many physicians administer two or three injections spaced about 1 month apart. Extrapolating from knee osteoarthritis data, we hypothesize that the duration of effects is 12 months or greater.

Data on safety and efficacy

As previously mentioned, PRP has become a popular modality in sports medicine to treat knee osteoarthritis,[47,48] tendonopathy,[44,45] ligament injury,[44,45] and muscle strain.[44,45] There are limited data on the utility of PRP for SIJ pain.

Ko et al. in 2017 published a case series of four patients with SIJ dysfunction. Each patient received two separate 10-mL injections into the posterior sacroiliac ligaments (not intraarticular) with ultrasound guidance. Patients were followed up at 1 and 4 years after the PRP injection. The results showed a statistically significant decrease in pain at 1 and 4 years after treatment. The patients also reported an improvement in their overall quality of life.[50]

A prospective study examined the efficacy of steroid versus PRP ultrasound-guided SIJ injections for chronic low back pain.[51] Participants in the steroid group received a methylprednisolone and lidocaine mixture and the PRP group received 3 mL leukocyte-free PRP with 0.5 mL calcium chloride. Patients were evaluated at 2, 4, and 6 weeks as well as 3 months after the injection. There was no statistical difference between the two groups at 2 and 4 weeks. However, at 6 weeks and 3 months, the PRP group had significantly lower intensity of pain compared to the steroid group. The researchers also observed a lasting effect in the PRP group: 90% of the patients in the PRP group were pain free at 3 months versus 25% of the patients in the steroid group.[51]

An additional case series of 10 patients in 2015 received fluoroscopy-guided SIJ injections using 4 mL PRP. At 3 months, all patients had improved and did not require any additional treatments for their SIJ pain for up to 6 months.[52]

The evidence is extremely limited for the efficacy of PRP for SIJ-related pain, and further RCTs are required.

PRP is a relatively safe procedure, with a low incidence (2–5%) of side effects.[45] The most common side effects reported are local tenderness and pain.[45,53] Neither of the case series mentioned earlier in this section reported any adverse events.[50,52] In the 2017 study, post-injection pain and stiffness had a higher incidence in the PRP group compared to the steroid group, but these side effects improved within 2 days.[51] Overall, PRP appears to have a good safety profile.

The discontinuation of nonsteroidal anti-inflammatory drugs (NSAIDs) is recommended to allow for the desired inflammatory response to develop. For this same reason, PRP should be delayed until approximately 6 weeks after corticosteroid injection in the same region.[54] Since PRP is from the patient's own blood, there is no risk of an allergic reaction to the injectant itself. Contraindications to PRP include low platelet count, low hemoglobin (<10 g/dL), platelet dysfunction, use of NSAIDs within 48 hours of the procedure, corticosteroid injection at the treatment site within 2 weeks of the procedure, corticosteroid by mouth or intravenously within 2 weeks of the procedure, septicemia, active infections, and active cancer.

Preparation and administration

Unfortunately, there is a wide variety of reported preparation protocols, with variables including platelet concentration, volume injected, addition of platelet activators, white blood cell concentration, neutrophil percentage, and concentration of red blood cells.[55] The general preparation of PRP is as follows.

Whole blood is drawn from the patient, and then sodium citrate, acid-citrate-dextrose, or ethylene diamine tetra-acetic acid is added to the whole blood to prevent clot formation.[56] It is then placed in a centrifuge to separate the red blood cells from the "buffy coat" and the platelet-poor plasma (Figure 9.3). The buffy coat is a thin white layer that is rich in platelets and contains leukocytes. A second centrifugation step is used to further separate the PRP from the platelet-poor plasma. Again, there is heterogeneity between studies on the use of the second centrifuge step. Calcium chloride can be added to the PRP to ensure platelet degranulation.[49,56] Some report adding calcium chloride during the second centrifuge step, and others report adding it prior to the isolated platelet-rich layer beforeadministration to the patient.[49,56] The variability of PRP preparations makes it difficult to elucidate the efficacy of PRP.

Autologous whole blood

Background

Autologous whole blood (WB) contains molecules to mediate inflammation, angiogenesis, and cell migration.[57] WB contains platelets that release growth factor to promote healing. The presence of red and white blood cells in autologous WB may confound the effectiveness of the platelet-derived growth factors.[58] Use of PRP has significantly increased in the past as opposed to WB, and the comparative efficacy between the two is controversial.

Pharmacology

Similar to PRP, WB contains platelets and growth factors thought to stimulate healing.[59-61] It is possible that injection of WB induces a healing cascade that may improve SIJ pain related to ligament laxity or degenerative arthritis.

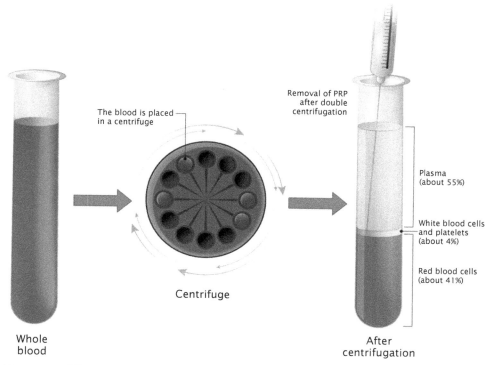

The blood is placed in a centrifuge

Removal of PRP after double centrifugation

Plasma (about 55%)

White blood cells and platelets (about 4%)

Red blood cells (about 41%)

Centrifuge

Whole blood

After centrifugation

FIGURE 9.3. PRP preparation process. Designua/Shutterstock.com

Data on safety and efficacy

While we do not have good data regarding the SIJ itself, a study evaluating tendinopathies at other locations documents improvement in pain and function at 4 weeks, with further improvement at 8 weeks.[60] Similarly, Edwards et al. report maximal benefit from the injection at 3 weeks on average.[61] Since it is thought to be regenerative, repeat injections can be performed. Intervals between WB injections are not well defined, but 4 to 8 weeks has been described.[61] With it taking up to 8 weeks for maximum benefit from the first injection, we recommend waiting at least 8 weeks for a repeat injection after the first treatment with WB, but these intervals can be decreased if need be for further injection therapy.

To the authors' knowledge, there are no published trials evaluating the use of autologous WB injections for SIJ pain. As previously discussed, there are limited data on the use of PRP for SIJ pain and the qualitative evidence has been assessed as Level IV (on a scale of Level I through V) using a qualitative modified approach to the grading of evidence based on WB best evidence synthesis.[62]

While we do not have studies focused on the SIJ, there are published data focusing on other inflammatory and degenerative musculoskeletal painful conditions that are of interest. A meta-analysis in 2019 evaluated the efficacy of autologous blood products versus corticosteroid injection to treat patients with plantar fasciitis.[63] Patients who received corticosteroid had a great reduction in pain than patients who received WB at 1.5 and 3 months after injection.[63]

An RCT comparing PRP to WB for the treatment of chronic lateral epicondylitis concluded that PRP may be slightly superior at 8 weeks after injection.[64] A study by Kazemi et al. demonstrated that a localized injection of WB had a larger therapeutic benefit than steroid injection for the treatment of tennis elbow.[60]

The main risks would be from the injection itself, to include bleeding, bruising, and infection. Patients can experience pain at the location of the injection, but this has been described as comparable to steroid injections.[61] It is important to maintain sterile technique with venous blood aspiration as well as injection into the SIJ to prevent infection.

Preparation and administration

Autologous WB is not altered for the injection. Some studies report mixing the WB with 1 mL 2% lidocaine or 0.5% bupivacaine,[61] but this is not necessary. Sterile technique is used throughout, to include the removal of venous blood. The volume for the SIJ is variable, but the authors recommend 3 mL for intraarticular injections and 5 mL for periarticular injections.

Hyaluronic acid

Background

Hyaluronic acid (HA), also known as hyaluronan, is a non-sulfated glycosaminoglycan. It is synthesized in the cellular plasma membrane as opposed to the Golgi apparatus, which makes it distinct from other glycosaminoglycans. HA has a large molecular weight about 7 million Daltons per molecule.[65] HA is a main component of extracellular matrix and is thought to contribute to tissue regeneration and angiogenesis and mediates the inflammatory response.[66] HA is used in many fields of medicine, including orthopedic surgery for osteoarthritis, ophthalmology for dry eyes, and aesthetic medicine for cosmetic fillers.[67]

Pharmacology

A systematic review in 2015 on the mechanism of action of HA for osteoarthritis of the knee found chondroprotection was the most common mechanism reported.[68] Intraarticular HA reduces chondrocyte apoptosis and increases chondrocyte proliferation.[69] This is thought to be mediated by HA binding with CD44.[68,69] HA has an anti-inflammatory property by suppressing IL-1beta.[70] Several studies have suggested HA lubricates the joint capsule in knee osteoarthritis, preventing further degeneration.[68] The anti-inflammatory effects and joint lubrication may be translated to the SIJ in future studies.

There are limited data on HA for SIJ pain. For knee osteoarthritis, onset of clinically meaningful results after intraarticular HA injection was 1 to 4 weeks and the effect lasted for 6 to 12 months.[71]

Data on safety and efficacy

A literature search for HA for SIJ produced one case series of four patients with SIJ syndrome. Each participant received three injections of Hylan GF 20 into the SIJ 2 weeks apart. At 12 and 16 weeks after the injections, patients reported 40% to 67% improvement on the visual analog scale.[72]

A systematic review and meta-analysis in 2012 showed that in patients with knee osteoarthritis, HA was associated with a small and clinically irrelevant benefit.[73] Patients also had an increased risk of adverse events.[73] Jevsevar et al. in 2015 performed a meta-analysis of double-blinded, sham-controlled trials and did not find clinically important differences of HA treatment over placebo.[74]

Further studies are warranted to further evaluate the clinical efficacy of HA for SIJ pain.

Overall, intraarticular HA has a favorable safety profile. The most common side effect with HA injection is injection site pain and swelling.[75] With any intraarticular injection, there is also a risk of infection. An unusual complication that has been observed after intraarticular knee injection is an acute post-injection flare also called pseudoseptic reaction.[76,77] Patients will present with an effusion within 1 week of the injection.[76,77] Joint effusion cultures are negative and have no crystals. It has also been reported that HA can result in pseudogout a few days after injection.[75] These adverse events have been reported for intraarticular knee HA injections. Unfortunately, there is no current evidence on HA injection adverse events for SIJ pain.

Preparation and administration

HA products are produced from either avian sources or biologic fermentation. The avian-derived molecules are thought to be a possible cause of adverse side effects. The molecular weight of HA products has also been shown to be a factor in the effectiveness of HA injections for osteoarthritis. High-molecular-weight HA products are more favorable than the low-molecular-weight HA products for knee osteoarthritis.[73]

Conclusion

The field broadly referred to as "regenerative medicine" comprises a wide range of biologic agents, including PRP, MSCs, and other products as well as non–biologic-based therapies such as prolotherapy and HA. This chapter has summarized the pharmacology, data on safety and efficacy, and information on preparation and administration of these products based on current evidence and best practice recommendations. The American Society of Interventional Pain Practice has offered guidelines for the use of biologic agents for low back pain including SIJ pain, summarizing the evidence as Level IV (of V) for the use of PRP for SIJ pain.[78] Overall there is a clear paucity of data clearly demonstrating the safety and efficacy of regenerative medicine in the treatment of SIJ-mediated pain. Nevertheless, SIJ-mediated pain in the setting of degenerative joint disease is considered to be similar to peripheral joint pain, for which the degree of evidence is much more robust. Many practitioners look to data regarding peripheral joints to discuss with the patients the risks versus benefits of considering regenerative medicine therapy for SIJ-mediated pain.

Cossu et al. are among several voices raising alarm over the rapidly expanding field of regenerative medicine and point out the widening gap between the optimism and hope of regenerative medicine therapies and the science supporting its efficacy in its wide range of purported applications.[79] The profit margin realized by some private clinics poses significant ethical concerns regarding the use of regenerative medicine, and governmental regulatory bodies have at times struggled to meet the pace of the expanding field. There is a qualitative difference between areas of research conducted under the regulation of IND with rigorously peer-reviewed published findings and the widespread commercialization of regenerative medicine products. The lack of evidence as demonstrated by high-quality RCTs supporting the safety and efficacy of regenerative medicine therapies for SIJ pain is clear, even though practitioners across the country offer this service to patients for relief of musculoskeletal pain. A balance must be struck between the paucity of evidence and scientific clarity regarding the mechanisms of regenerative medicine and the hope offered to patients suffering from debilitating pain leading to compromised function. High-quality RCTs are needed to evaluate the effectiveness of regenerative medicine for SIJ-related pain, ideally with the close support and guidance of the FDA to offer clear structure for operating within an IND and publishing clinical results using validated outcome measures.

References

1. Cohen SP, Chen Y, Neufeld NJ. Sacroiliac joint pain: A comprehensive review of epidemiology, diagnosis and treatment. Expert Rev Neurother. 2013;13(1):99–116.
2. Cohen SP. Epidemics, evolution, and sacroiliac joint pain. Reg Anesth Pain Med. 2007;32(1):3–6.
3. Mooney V. Prolotherapy at the fringe of medical care, or is it the frontier? Spine J. 2003;3(4):253–254.
4. Schultz LW. A treatment for subluxation of the temporomandibular joint. JAMA. 1937;109(13):1032–1035.
5. Rabago D, Slattengren A, Zgierska A. Prolotherapy in primary care practice. Prim Care. 2010;37(1):65–80.
6. Chuang CW, Hung SK, Pan PT, et al. Diagnosis and interventional pain management options for sacroiliac joint pain. Ci Ji Yi Xue Za Zhi. 2019;31(4):207–210.
7. Banks AR. A rationale for prolotherapy. J Orthop Med. 1991;13(3):54–59.
8. Linetsky FS, Trescot AM, Wiederholz MH. Regenerative injection therapy. In Sackheim K (Ed.), Pain management and palliative care. Springer, 2015.
9. Rabago D, Nourani B. Prolotherapy for osteoarthritis and tendinopathy: A descriptive review. Curr Rheumatol Rep. 2017;19(6):34.
10. DeChellis DM, Cortzaao MH. Regenerative medicine in the field of pain medicine: Prolotherapy, platelet-rich plasma therapy, and stem cell therapy—theory and evidence. Tech Reg Anesth Pain Manage. 2011;15(2):74–80.
11. Hauser RA, Maddela HS, Alderman D, et al. *Journal of Prolotherapy* International Medical Editorial Board consensus statement on the use of prolotherapy for musculoskeletal pain. J Prolother. 2011;3(4):744–764.
12. Di Paolo S, Gesualdo L, Ranieri E, et al. High glucose concentration induces the overexpression of transforming growth factor-beta through the activation of a platelet-derived growth factor loop in human mesangial cells. Am J Pathol. 1996;149(6):2095–2106.
13. Jensen KT, Rabago DP, Best TM, et al. Early inflammatory response of knee ligaments to prolotherapy in a rat model. J Orthop Res. 2008;26(6):816–823.

14. Schwarzer AC, Aprill CN, Bogduk N. The sacroiliac joint in chronic low back pain. Spine. 1995;20(1):31–37.

15. Cusi M, Saunders J, Hungerford B, et al. The use of prolotherapy in the sacroiliac joint. Br J Sports Med. 2010;44(2):100–104.

16. Hoffman MD, Agnish V. Functional outcome from sacroiliac joint prolotherapy in patients with sacroiliac joint instability. Complement Ther Med. 2018;37:64–68.

17. Yelland MJ, Mar C, Pirozzo S, et al. Prolotherapy injections for chronic low-back pain. Cochrane Database Syst Rev. 2004(2):CD004059.

18. Rabago D, Best TM, Beamsley M, et al. A systematic review of prolotherapy for chronic musculoskeletal pain. Clin J Sports Med. 2005;15(5):376–380.

19. Aneja A, Karas SG, Weinhold PS, et al. Suture plication, thermal shrinkage, and sclerosing agents: Effects on rat patellar tendon length and biomechanical strength. Am J Sports Med. 2005;33(11):1729–1734.

20. Reeves KD, Hassanein KM. Long-term effects of dextrose prolotherapy for anterior cruciate ligament laxity. Altern Ther Health Med. 2003;9(3):58–62.

21. Kim WM, Lee HG, Jeong CW, et al. A randomized controlled trial of intra-articular prolotherapy versus steroid injection for sacroiliac joint pain. J Altern Complement Med. 2010;16(12):1285–1290.

22. Gall EA. The cytological identity and interrelation of mesenchymal cells of lymphoid tissue. Ann N Y Acad Sci. 1958;73(1):120–130.

23. Mahla RS. Stem cells applications in regenerative medicine and disease therapeutics. Int J Cell Biol. 2016;2016:6940283.

24. Dominici M, Le Blanc K, Mueller I, et al. Minimal criteria for defining multipotent mesenchymal stromal cells. The International Society for Cellular Therapy position statement. Cytotherapy. 2006;8(4):315–317.

25. Samsonraj RM, Raghunath M, Nurcombe V, et al. Concise review: Multifaceted characterization of human mesenchymal stem cells for use in regenerative medicine. Stem Cells Transl Med. 2017;6(12):2173–2185.

26. Witwer KW, Van Balkom BWM, Bruno S, et al. Defining mesenchymal stromal cell (MSC)-derived small extracellular vesicles for therapeutic applications. J Extracell Vesicles. 2019;8(1):1609206.

27. de Souza LE, Malta TM, Kashima Haddad S, et al. Mesenchymal stem cells and pericytes: To what extent are they related? Stem Cells Dev. 2016;25(24):1843–1852.

28. Esteves CL, Donadeu FX. Pericytes and their potential in regenerative medicine across species. Cytometry A. 2018;93(1):50–59.

29. Robinson PG, Murray IR, West CC, et al. Reporting of mesenchymal stem cell preparation protocols and composition: A systematic review of the clinical orthopaedic literature. Am J Sports Med. 2019;47(4):991–1000.

30. Murphy MB, Moncivais K, Caplan AI. Mesenchymal stem cells: Environmentally responsive therapeutics for regenerative medicine. Exp Mol Med. 2013;45(11):e54.

31. Caplan AI. New MSC: MSCs as pericytes are sentinels and gatekeepers. J Orthop Res. 2017;35(6):1151–1159.

32. Desai MJ, Mansfield JT, Robinson DM, et al. Regenerative medicine for axial and radicular spine-related pain: A narrative review. Pain Pract. 2020;20(4):437–453.

33. Pettine KA, Suzuki RK, Sand TT, et al. Autologous bone marrow concentrate intradiscal injection for the treatment of degenerative disc disease with three-year follow-up. Int Orthop. 2017;41(10):2097–2103.

34. Orozco L, Soler R, Morera C, et al. Intervertebral disc repair by autologous mesenchymal bone marrow cells: A pilot study. Transplantation. 2011;92(7):822–828.

35. Haufe SM, Mork AR. Intradiscal injection of hematopoietic stem cells in an attempt to rejuvenate the intervertebral discs. Stem Cells Dev. 2006;15(1):136–137.

36. Kubrova E, D'Souza RS, Hunt CL, et al. Injectable biologics: What is the evidence? Am J Phys Med Rehabil. 2020;99(10):950–960.

37. Ha CW, Park YB, Kim SH, et al. Intra-articular mesenchymal stem cells in osteoarthritis of the knee: A systematic review of clinical outcomes and evidence of cartilage repair. Arthroscopy. 2019;35(1):277–288.

38. Gentile P, Calabrese C, De Angelis B, et al. Impact of the different preparation methods to obtain human adipose-derived stromal vascular fraction cells (AD-SVFs) and human adipose-derived mesenchymal stem cells (AD-MSCs): Enzymatic digestion versus mechanical centrifugation. Int J Mol Sci. 2019;20(21):5471.

39. Regulatory Considerations for Human Cells, Tissues, and Cellular and Tissue-Based Products: Minimal Manipulation and Homologous Use. 2020:25.

40. Hernigou J, Picard L, Alves A, et al. Understanding bone safety zones during bone marrow aspiration from the iliac crest: The sector rule. Int Orthop. 2014;38(11):2377–2384.

41. Shapiro SA, Arthurs JR. Bone marrow aspiration for regenerative orthopedic intervention: Technique with ultrasound guidance for needle placement. Regen Med. 2017;12(8):917–928.

42. D'Souza RS, Li L, Leng S, et al. A three-dimensional computed tomography study to determine the ideal method for fluoroscopically-guided bone marrow aspiration from the iliac crest. Bosn J Basic Med Sci. 2020 [online before print].

43. Kubrova E, Su M, Galeano-Garces C, et al. Differences in cytotoxicity of lidocaine, ropivacaine, bupivacaine on the viability and metabolic activity of human adipose-derived mesenchymal stem cells. Am J Phys Med Rehabil. 2021;100(1):82–91.

44. Moraes VY, Lenza M, Tamaoki MJ, et al. Platelet-rich therapies for musculoskeletal soft tissue injuries. Cochrane Database Syst Rev. 2014(4):CD010071.

45. Filardo G, Kon E, Della Villa S, et al. Use of platelet-rich plasma for the treatment of refractory jumper's knee. Int Orthop. 2010;34(6):909–915.

46. Hsu WK, Mishra A, Rodeo SR, et al. Platelet-rich plasma in orthopaedic applications: Evidence-based recommendations for treatment. J Am Acad Orthop Surg. 2013;21(12):739–748.

47. Andia I, Maffulli N. Platelet-rich plasma for managing pain and inflammation in osteoarthritis. Nat Rev Rheumatol. 2013;9(12):721–730.

48. Laudy AB, Bakker EW, Rekers M, et al. Efficacy of platelet-rich plasma injections in osteoarthritis of the knee: A systematic review and meta-analysis. Br J Sports Med. 2015;49(10):657–672.

49. Foster TE, Puskas BL, Mandelbaum BR, et al. Platelet-rich plasma: From basic science to clinical applications. Am J Sports Med. 2009;37(11):2259–2272.

50. Marx RE. Platelet-rich plasma (PRP): What is PRP and what is not PRP? Implant Dent. 2001;10(4):225–228.

51. Ko GD, Mindra S, Lawson GE, et al. Case series of ultrasound-guided platelet-rich plasma injections for sacroiliac joint dysfunction. J Back Musculoskelet Rehabil. 2017;30(2):363–370.

52. Singla V, Batra YK, Bharti N, et al. Steroid vs. platelet-rich plasma in ultrasound-guided sacroiliac joint injection for chronic low back pain. Pain Pract. 2017;17(6):782–791.

53. Peerbooms JC, Sluimer J, Bruijn DJ, et al. Positive effect of an autologous platelet concentrate in lateral epicondylitis in a double-blind randomized controlled trial: Platelet-rich plasma versus corticosteroid injection with a 1-year follow-up. Am J Sports Med. 2010;38(2):255–262.

54. Glynn LG, Mustafa A, Casey M, et al. Platelet-rich plasma (PRP) therapy for knee arthritis: A feasibility study in primary care. Pilot Feasibility Stud. 2018;4:93.

55. Rossi LA, Murray IR, Chu CR, et al. Classification systems for platelet-rich plasma. Bone Joint J. 2019;101-B(8):891–896.

56. Le ADK, Enweze L, DeBaun MR, et al. Platelet-rich plasma. Clin Sports Med. 2019;38(1):17–44.

57. Vannini F, Di Matteo B, Filardo G, et al. Platelet-rich plasma for foot and ankle pathologies: A systematic review. Foot Ankle Surg. 2014;20(1):2–9.

58. Kampa RJ, Connell DA. Treatment of tendinopathy: Is there a role for autologous whole blood and platelet rich plasma injection? Int J Clin Pract. 2010;64(13):1813–1823.

59. Mishra A, Pavelko T. Treatment of chronic elbow tendinosis with buffered platelet-rich plasma. Am J Sports Med. 2006;34(11):1774–1778.

60. Kazemi M, Azma K, Tavana B, et al. Autologous blood versus corticosteroid local injection in the short-term treatment of lateral elbow tendinopathy: A randomized clinical trial of efficacy. Am J Phys Med Rehabil. 2010;89(8):660–667.

61. Edwards SG, Calandruccio JH. Autologous blood injections for refractory lateral epicondylitis. J Hand Surg Am. 2003;28(2):272–278.

62. Sanapati J, Manchikanti L, Atluri S, et al. Do regenerative medicine therapies provide long-term relief in chronic low back pain: A systematic review and metaanalysis. Pain Physician. 2018;21(6):515–540.

63. Chen YJ, Wu YC, Tu YK, et al. Autologous blood-derived products compared with corticosteroids for treatment of plantar fasciopathy: A systematic review and meta-analysis. Am J Phys Med Rehabil. 2019;98(5):343–352.

64. Raeissadat SA, Rayegani SM, Hassanabadi H, et al. Is platelet-rich plasma superior to whole blood in the management of chronic tennis elbow: One year randomized clinical trial. BMC Sports Sci Med Rehabil. 2014;6:12.

65. Fraser JR, Laurent TC, Laurent UB. Hyaluronan: Its nature, distribution, functions and turnover. J Intern Med. 1997;242(1):27–33.

66. Shaharudin A, Aziz Z. Effectiveness of hyaluronic acid and its derivatives on chronic wounds: A systematic review. J Wound Care. 2016;25(10):585–592.

67. Salwowska NM, Bebenek KA, Zadlo DA, et al. Physiochemical properties and application of hyaluronic acid: A systematic review. J Cosmet Dermatol. 2016;15(4):520–526.

68. Altman RD, Manjoo A, Fierlinger A, et al. The mechanism of action for hyaluronic acid treatment in the osteoarthritic knee: A systematic review. BMC Musculoskelet Disord. 2015;16:321.

69. Elmorsy S, Funakoshi T, Sasazawa F, et al. Chondroprotective effects of high-molecular-weight cross-linked hyaluronic acid in a rabbit knee osteoarthritis model. Osteoarthritis Cartilage. 2014;22(1):121–127.

70. Sasaki A, Sasaki K, Konttinen YT, et al. Hyaluronate inhibits the interleukin-1beta-induced expression of matrix metalloproteinase (MMP)-1 and MMP-3 in human synovial cells. Tohoku J Exp Med. 2004;204(2):99–107.

71. Legre-Boyer V. Viscosupplementation: Techniques, indications, results. Orthop Traumatol Surg Res. 2015;101(1 Suppl):S101–S108.

72. Srejic U, Calvillo O, Kabakibou K. Viscosupplementation: A new concept in the treatment of sacroiliac joint syndrome: A preliminary report of four cases. Reg Anesth Pain Med. 1999;24(1):84–88.

73. Rutjes AW, Juni P, da Costa BR, et al. Viscosupplementation for osteoarthritis of the knee: A systematic review and meta-analysis. Ann Intern Med. 2012;157(3):180–191.

74. Jevsevar D, Donnelly P, Brown GA, et al. Viscosupplementation for osteoarthritis of the knee: A systematic review of the evidence. J Bone Joint Surg Am. 2015;97(24):2047–2060.

75. Hamburger MI, Lakhanpal S, Mooar PA, et al. Intra-articular hyaluronans: A review of product-specific safety profiles. Semin Arthritis Rheum. 2003;32(5):296–309.

76. Puttick MP, Wade JP, Chalmers A, et al. Acute local reactions after intraarticular Hylan for osteoarthritis of the knee. J Rheumatol. 1995;22(7):1311–1314.

77. Pullman-Mooar S, Mooar P, Sieck M, et al. Are there distinctive inflammatory flares after Hylan G-f 20 intraarticular injections? J Rheumatol. 2002;29(12):2611–2614.

78. Navani A, Manchikanti L, Albers SL, et al. Responsible, safe, and effective use of biologics in the management of low back pain: American Society of Interventional Pain Physicians (ASIPP) guidelines. Pain Physician. 2019;22(1s):S1–S74.

79. Cossu G, Birchall M, Brown T, et al. Lancet Commission: Stem cells and regenerative medicine. Lancet. 2018;391(10123):883–910.

10

Imaging techniques for sacroiliac joint injections

Jacqueline Weisbein

Introduction

Sacroiliac joint (SIJ) injections can be used for both diagnostic and therapeutic purposes. One subset of therapeutic injections includes regenerative medicine. This can include a variety of techniques, such as injections guided by computed tomography (CT), fluoroscopy, and ultrasound. Absolute contraindications to injections include local malignancy and infection. Relative contraindications include coagulopathy, pregnancy (depending on the type of imaging), systemic infection, a septic joint, or osteomyelitis.

CT-guided SIJ procedure

In a study of 71 CT-guided injections of the SIJ, Pulisetti et al. concluded that CT guidance is the most precise method for confirming diagnostic injections.[1] Typically, the first step is to place the patient prone on the table and perform a preliminary single-slice CT scan of the SIJs. The skin is prepared and draped in meticulous sterile fashion. Then, using a low-dose/pulse technique, the position of entry is marked approximately 1 cm above the lower end of the articular space. The sacroiliac cleft is then approached using a freehand technique.[2] The joint space is typically confirmed by injecting at least 1 to 3 mL of nonionic contrast medium (Ioversol, Optiray, Covidien, Mansfield, MA, USA).[3] The injectate is then placed (Figure 10.1).

The most common complications noted with CT-guided procedures, other than the typical noted complications, are transient reactions such as vasovagal reactions.[4] By maintaining sterile/aseptic technique, complications are limited other than radiation exposure.

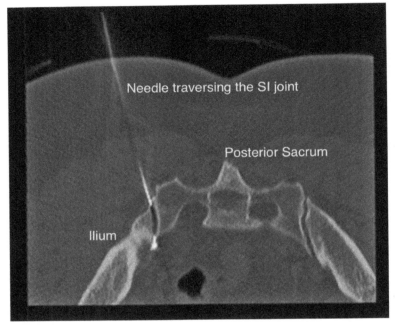

Needle traversing the SI joint

Posterior Sacrum

Ilium

FIGURE 10.1. SIJ injection under CT guidance.

Fluoroscopy-guided SIJ procedure

Similar to intraarticular injections with steroids, this procedure should be performed in a sterile environment in either the office or an outpatient surgical center. The patient is placed in a prone position on a radiolucent table. Typically, a pillow is placed under the lower portion of the abdomen to assist in visualization. After sterile preparation and draping, the C-arm is brought into the field. The image intensifier should then be rotated in a contralateral oblique fashion anywhere from 10 to 20 degrees to help visualize the joint space. Then, radiopaque contrast can be administered to outline the joint space. Many using fluoroscopic guidance will confirm the view without using contrast in anteroposterior (AP), oblique, and lateral views under fluoroscopy (Figure 10.2).[5]

After the needle location is confirmed, the injectate is placed. An average of 4 to 6 mL of injectate is used, half intraarticular and the other periarticular. The goal is to infiltrate the joint as well as the interosseous ligament. Of note, Khuba et al. suggested that the oblique angulation may be unnecessary and that one might enter the lower part of the posterior joint using an AP image alone.[6] Chauhan et al. demonstrated in a randomized controlled study that it allowed for access to the joint with shorter fluoroscopy times.[7]

Complications from specific injectates are described in Chapter 9. However, complications from this type of injection tend to be nonexistent, as reported by Navani et al.,[5] or limited to increased pain in approximately 15% to 30% of patients.[8] Maugars et al. also described a brief increase in pain after the injection, as well as transient perineal anesthesia or a temporary sciatalgia after injection.[9] Although rare, complications of septic arthritis can occur in

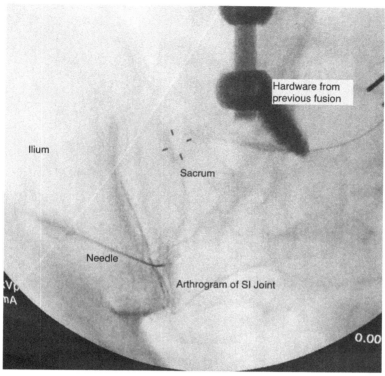

FIGURE 10.2. Arthrogram of the left SIJ demonstrating optimal contrast pattern. *Source:* Courtesy of J. Weisbein, DO

patients with increased risk factors such as diabetes mellitus, presence of prosthetic material, localized infections, older age, and use of immunosuppressive medications.[10] Using the lateral view can help prevent inadvertent administration of the injection into the pelvic viscera.[11]

Ultrasound-guided SIJ procedure

Hartung et al. described the ultrasound-guided injection in a method that has been adopted by many. The patient is placed in the prone position on the table with a pillow under the pelvis. The feet are then internally rotated with an inversion to make the joint more easily accessible. The skin is prepared in a meticulous sterile fashion and then, using an ultrasound with a linear array transducer in a 2.5- to 8.0-MHz frequency with the field of view set at 44 mm, scanning and visualization of the SIJ cleft are performed (Figure 10.3).[12] The SIJ can be observed as a hypoechoic cleft area between the two echogenic lines of the sacrum and iliac bone.[13] Then, the needle is advanced into the joint space. Saunders et al. described a modification of Hartung's technique that targets the synovial portion of the joint with the goal of injecting into and around the dorsal interosseous ligament while avoiding the synovial part of the joint. Typically, the dorsal interosseous ligament is found at the S1–S2 level, which is where the therapeutic injection should be administered.[14]

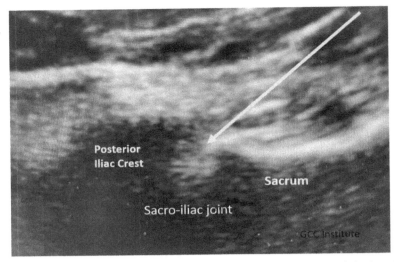

FIGURE 10.3. SIJ injection under ultrasound guidance. The needle is traveling from medial to lateral with local prior the placement of the spinal needle. *Source:* Image used with permission from George Chang Chien, DO

Complications such as infection are a potential issue with any injection if appropriate sterile technique is not used. Serious complications of ultrasound-guided intraarticular injections, like advancement of the needle into the retropelvic area, are uncommon.[15] It seems that with ultrasound-guided injections, accuracy of the placement is less likely to be intraarticular.[16] However, Hartung et al.'s previously referenced work indicates that periarticular injectate administration can still be efficacious with regard to steroid. As previously noted, many administer platelet-rich plasma both intraarticularly and periarticularly, so this should not pose a complication. One of the most interesting differences is that the procedural time is much longer with ultrasound than other modalities, but this is likely related to other variables.[17] With increased experience and progression of skill, extravasation into the retroperitoneal space can be reduced and the amount of time per injection can be decreased.[14] Conversely, visualization with ultrasound of any possible extraarticular spread when caused by extraarticular needle placement can allow the needle to be redirected to achieve intraarticular injection.[18]

Conclusion

Injection techniques for the SIJ vary based on the practitioner's training and experience. In contrast to injectates like corticosteroids, typically the injectates in regenerative medicine are derived from the patient's own blood. Therefore, the risks for patients are often similar to transfusion reactions or allergic or immune reactions. If products are from the patient's own body, there are no risks associated with the injection or drug interaction other than the possibility of breaking sterile technique or administration into a structure and damaging that.

References

1. Pulisetti D, Ebraheim NA. CT-guided sacroiliac joint injections. J Spinal Disord. 1999;12(4):310–312.
2. Althoff CE, Bollow M, Feist E, et al. CT-guided corticosteroid injection of the sacroiliac joints: Quality assurance and standardized prospective evaluation of long-term effectiveness over six months. Clin Rheumatol. 2015;34(6):1079–1084. doi:10.1007/s10067-015-2937-7. PMID: 25896531.
3. Sahin O, Harman A, Akgun R, Tuncay I. An intraarticular sacroiliac steroid injection under the guidance of computed tomography for relieving sacroiliac joint pain: A clinical outcome study with two years of follow-up. Turk J Rheumatol 2012;27:165–173.
4. Kennedy DJ, Schneider B, Casey E, et al. Vasovagal rates in fluoroscopically guided interventional procedures: A study of over 8,000 injections. Pain Med. 2013;14(12):1854–1859.
5. Navani A, Gupta D. Role of intra-articular platelet-rich plasma in sacroiliac joint pain. Tech Reg Anesth Pain Manag. 2015;19:54–59.
6. Khuba S, Agarwal A, Gautam S, et al. Fluoroscopic sacroiliac joint injection: Is oblique angulation really necessary? Pain Physician. 2016;19:E1135–E1138.
7. Chauhan G, Hehar P, Loomba V, Upadhyay A. A randomized controlled trial of fluoroscopically-guided sacroiliac joint injections: A comparison of the posteroanterior and classical oblique techniques. Neurospine. 2019;16(2):317–324. doi:10.14245/ns.1836122.061
8. Cheng J, Abdi S. Complications of joint, tendon, and muscle injections. Tech Reg Anesth Pain Manag. 2007;11(3):141–147. doi:10.1053/j.trap.2007.05.006
9. Maugars Y, Mathis C, Berthelot JM, et al. Assessment of the efficacy of sacroiliac corticosteroid injections in spondylarthropathies: A double-blind study. Br J Rheumatol. 1996;35:767–770.
10. Charalambous CP, Tryfonidis M, Sadiq S, et al. Septic arthritis following intra-articular steroid injection of the knee: A survey of current practice regarding antiseptic technique used during intra-articular steroid injection of the knee. Clin Rheumatol 2003;22:386–390.
11. Kothari G, Berkwits L, Batson JP, Furman MB. Sacroiliac intraarticular joint injections, posterior approach, inferior entry. In HS Smith (Ed.), Current therapy in pain. Saunders, 2009.
12. Hartung W, Ross CJ, Straub R, et al. Ultrasound-guided sacroiliac joint injection in patients with established sacroiliitis: Precise IA injection verified by MRI scanning does not predict clinical outcome. Rheumatology. 2010;49:1479–1482.
13. Pekkafahli MZ, Kiralp MZ, Basekim CC, et al. Sacroiliac joint injections performed with sonographic guidance. J Ultrasound Med. 2003;22:553–559.
14. Saunders J, Cusi M, Hackett L, Van der Wall H. An exploration of ultrasound-guided therapeutic injection of the dorsal interosseous ligaments of the sacroiliac joint for mechanical dysfunction of the joint. JSM Pain Manag. 2016;1:1003–1007.
15. Jee H, Lee JH, Park KD, et al. Ultrasound-guided versus fluoroscopy-guided sacroiliac joint intraarticular injections in the noninflammatory sacroiliac joint dysfunction: A prospective, randomized, single-blinded study. Arch Phys Med Rehabil. 2014;95(2):330–337. doi:10.1016/j.apmr.2013.09.021. PMID: 24121083.
16. Wu L, Tafti D, Varacallo M. Sacroiliac joint injection. StatPearls, 2020. https://www.ncbi.nlm.nih.gov/books/NBK513245/
17. Soneji N, Bhatia A, Seib R, et al. Comparison of fluoroscopy and ultrasound guidance for sacroiliac joint injection in patients with chronic low back pain. Pain Pract. 2016;16:537–544.
18. Perry JM, Colberg RE, Dault SL, et al. A cadaveric study assessing the accuracy of ultrasound-guided sacroiliac joint injections. PM R. 2016;8(12):1168–1172.

Peripheral nerve stimulation for the sacroiliac joint

11

Patient selection and instruments used for peripheral nerve stimulation of the sacroiliac joint

Jessica Jameson

Patient selection

Peripheral nerve stimulation (PNS) has been shown to be efficacious in several chronic pain conditions. PNS is different from field stimulation in that there is a target peripheral nerve. This is an important distinction. Case reports over the previous decade have indicated that PNS can be useful in treating sacroiliac joint (SIJ) pain.[1-4]

When considering PNS as a potential treatment option for the SIJ, it is important to understand the peripheral nerves that supply the joint itself. This allows for a better understanding of the location and technique used to perform a diagnostic peripheral nerve block.

The medial cluneal nerve (MCN) is a purely sensory nerve that is made up of four to six branches. The pain emanating from this nerve is typically located in the lower lumbar area and buttocks. The MCN originates from the dorsal rami of S1–S4.[5] It passes below and sandwiches the long posterior sacroiliac ligament (LPSL) between the posterior superior iliac spine (PSIS) and the posterior inferior iliac spine and courses over the iliac crest to the buttocks.[6,7] In patients with low back and buttock pain, the MCN must be considered in the differential.

Pain due to MCN entrapment may be treated as SIJ pain and may respond to treatments aimed at the SIJ since the joint is innervated by the MCN. Although SIJ pain remains a controversial subject, it is thought to cause 15% to 30% of low back pain cases and is often associated with buttock to lower extremity symptoms.[8] There are no definitive medical history or physical examination findings that are consistently capable of identifying SIJ pain.[9] The physical examination tests, such as the Patrick test or the Gaenslen test, have low positive predictive value.[8] Radiologic imaging contributes little to the diagnosis; in fact, SIJ pain is typically a clinical diagnosis.[9] Fluoroscopically guided SIJ injections or blocks can solidify the diagnosis.[8] Fortin et al.[10] analyzed contrast extravasation patterns during 76 SIJ arthrograms by using computed tomography and found dorsal leakage around the LPSL in 18 cases (24%) and dorsal leakage into the S1 foramen in six (8%). The LPSL is a significant posterior ligamentous structure that resists shearing of the SIJ and certainly can be a potential pain generator in and of itself.

Murakami et al.[11] compared the effect of injections into the intraarticular space and periarticular region around the LPSL in patients with SIJ pain. The injection around the LPSL was effective in all 25 patients, whereas the intraarticular injection was effective in only nine out of 25 patients (36%). Furthermore, all 16 patients without pain relief after the intraarticular injection reported almost complete pain relief after injection around the LPSL. Fortin et al.[12] stated that SIJ patients could localize their pain with one finger, and the area pointed to was immediately inferomedial to the PSIS within 1 cm. Murakami et al.[11] observed a positive effect with periarticular SIJ block in 18 out of 25 patients who indicated the main site of pain within 2 cm of the PSIS. These results suggest that SIJ pain can originate from the LPSL as well as from the joint itself.

Lower back pain due to MCN entrapment is also affected by lumbar movement; in 82% of patients it elicited leg symptoms[5] and was aggravated by short and long periods of standing, lumbar flexion, rolling, prolonged sitting, and especially walking.[5] These symptoms are also similar to those of patients with lumbar disease. Therefore, a differential diagnosis must be made. In the presence of MCN entrapment, a Tinel-like sign is found 35 mm caudal to the PSIS at a slightly lateral point at the edge of the iliac crest, an area that corresponds with the nerve compression zone.[5] These patients report numbness and radiating pain in the MCN area upon trigger-point compression. This is a key diagnostic finding. The MCN must not be forgotten as a cause of neuropathic lower back pain (Box 11.1).

In broad terms, PNS is recommended when a patient's symptoms are refractory to conventional interventions such as physical therapy, medications, transcutaneous electrical nerve stimulation (TENS), and nerve blocks or injections. It is important to consider correctable pathologies prior to considering PNS. These can be excluded using diagnostic and imaging studies.

BOX 11.1. Diagnostic criteria for MCN symptoms

1 Low back pain involving the buttocks
2 Symptoms exacerbated by lumbar movement or posture
3 Tenderness to palpation approximately 35 mm caudal to the posterior superior iliac spine
4 Patients report numbness and radiating pain in the MCN area when the trigger point is compressed
5 Symptom relief by MCN block

Additionally, as with all neuromodulation techniques, psychological evaluation may be undertaken to identify factors that may impact the outcome, such as secondary gain and mood or personality disorders. A number of studies have examined psychological variables associated with response to pain treatment. In general, a handful of risk factors have been identified that correlate with greater risk for unsuccessful outcomes from pain treatment, including pain chronicity and duration, psychological distress, pain-related catastrophizing, a history of abuse or trauma, nicotine use and substance abuse history, poor social support, and significant cognitive deficits.[13] In general, patients with psychiatric comorbidity and high levels of distress, particularly psychopathology/extreme emotionality, have poor responses to treatment.[14-17] It is widely recognized that patients with chronic pain frequently report depression, anxiety, irritability, history of physical/sexual abuse, a personal and family history of mood disorder, and other risk factors for deleterious pain-related outcomes.[15] In chronic pain clinic populations, 50% to 80% of patients with chronic pain had signs of psychopathology,[16] making this the most prevalent comorbidity in these patients. This underscores the importance of obtaining a psychological evaluation for those being considered for spinal cord stimulation therapy.

The criteria for patient selection are as follows:

1. Pain consistent with the sensory distribution of a single peripheral nerve
2. A positive diagnostic peripheral nerve block
3. The patient is free of major psychological or psychiatric disease
4. Ability to use and operate the device

These selection criteria represent a consensus based on the clinical experience and suggestions of multiple published studies. There are, however, no published studies that show any predictive value for diagnostic peripheral nerve blocks or the efficacy of a TENS unit on PNS success.[18]

The contraindications for the use of PNS relate to the surgical risk and include (1) coagulopathy, (2) infection at the surgical site, (3) psychiatric illness, (4) a failed diagnostic block, and (5) complete sensory loss. Those contraindications mainly apply to permanent PNS implants, and some are relative (it all depends on the risk vs. benefit). When counseling patients about the risks of the procedures, it is important to include a discussion on infection, nerve damage, electrode migration, mechanical failure (including disconnection of hardware), failure to provide adequate stimulation or pain relief, pain, and cosmetic concerns.

As with any interventional technique, concerns about anticoagulation status arise. The American Society of Regional Anesthesia and Pain Medicine, in coordination with the North American Neuromodulation Society, and others have provided guidelines on the procedural risk and recommendations for anticoagulants. Table 11.1 describes the risk stratification accompanied by the types of pain procedures typically performed. PNS falls into a low risk category for bleeding complications. As such, the risk of complications from stopping a blood thinner before the procedure may outweigh the risk of the procedure itself. The Society does note that patients at a high risk of bleeding (e.g., old age, history of

TABLE 11.1 Classification of various pain procedures according to risk if performed in patients taking anticoagulants

Classification	Pain procedure
High risk	Spinal cord stimulation, dorsal root ganglion stimulation, percutaneous decompression laminotomy, intrathecal catheter, vertebral augmentation, epiduroscopy
Intermediate risk	Epidural injections, transforaminal, cervical facet/MBNB/RFA, intradiscal procedures, sympathetic blocks, trigeminal blocks
Low risk	Peripheral nerve stimulation, peripheral joints, trigger points, sacroiliac joint injection, thoracic and lumbar facet/MBNB/RFA, pocket revision

From the American Society for Regional Anesthesia[19]

bleeding tendency, concurrent use of other anticoagulants, liver cirrhosis, advanced liver or renal disease) undergoing low- or intermediate-risk procedures should be treated as being at intermediate or high risk, respectively.

Instruments used

Neuromodulation devices comprise several distinct components that are consistent across a variety of manufacturers. The electrical energy is imparted to the target using small metal contacts arranged on a lead or electrode. These leads come in various shapes and sizes. The power used to run these devices comes from an implantable pulse generator (IPG) or an external generator. In the setting of an external generator, the system uses radiofrequency (RF) coupling that can deliver high-power complex stimulation. RF coupling also provides ease in replenishing this power supply as most external generators are powered by regular household batteries. RF generators do, however, require significantly more patient participation (powering, changing stimulation, etc.) than IPGs. IPG systems have limited internal battery power and therefore must be replaced every several years. This depends on the system usage, the battery size, and the stimulation parameters the patient uses.[20]

To place the electrode, an introducer is required. This introducer is often in the form of a Tuohy needle. This allows the skin to be entered and the lead to be placed through the needle once at the target nerve location. To identify landmarks and/or nerve location, ultrasound or radiographic guidance is needed. Once the lead has been placed, it is typically anchored to the underlying fascia using synthetic, nonabsorbable suture such as polyester (Ethibond), polypropylene (Prolene), or nylon (Ethilon) (Figure 11.1). Nonabsorbable sutures retain most of their tensile strength after 60 days.

Next, a pocket is created for the receiver. Tools used to do this can include a scalpel and Metzenbaum scissors versus blunt finger dissection. A tunneling device is then used to bring the lead into the created pocket. This is typically a long metal device with a plastic tube on the outside.

After irrigation, the wounds are closed with absorbable sutures. These are used to decrease dead space and to encourage subcutaneous wound approximation in deep layers

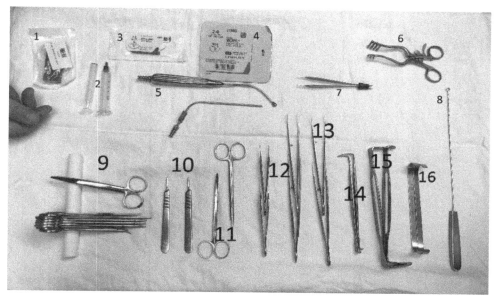

FIGURE 11.1. Tray setup. This is an example of surgical supplies commonly used for spinal cord stimulator implants but can vary based on different practice settings. 1: needle holder; 2: loss of resistance syringe; 3: anchor suture; 4: deep closure suture; 5: irrigation; 6: Weitlaner retractor; 7: bipolar diathermy; 8: radiopaque marker; 9: Mayo (suture) scissors; 10: scalpel handles; 11: tenotomy scissors; 12: tissue forceps; 13: Gerald tissue forceps; 14: Senn retractors; 15: Army-Navy retractors; 16: Farabeuf retractors.

prior to superficial skin closure. Superficial skin closure often involves staples or monofilament absorbable suture such as poliglecaprone (Monocryl) with or without Steri-Strips or adhesive for reinforcement. There is conflicting evidence about an increased risk for infection with staples. As such, the choice of suture or staples for superficial skin closure is left to the surgeon. Neither approach has been shown to be superior in terms of scar outcome or infection rates.[21,22]

The Neuromodulation Appropriateness Consensus Committee guidelines provide a helpful framework for considering best evidence–based practice for reducing infection risk, and all implanters should refer to this reference.[23] As technology advances, the size and difficulty of placing peripheral nerve stimulators, and thereby the risk, will decrease. This will allow for better stimulation and an increased ability to treat more patients.

References

1. Guentchev M, Preuss C, Rink R, et al. Technical note: Treatment of sacroiliac joint pain with peripheral nerve stimulation. Neuromodulation. 2015;18(5):392–396. doi:10.1111/ner.12255. PMID: 25354279.
2. Guentchev M, Preuss C, Rink R, et al. Long-term reduction of sacroiliac joint pain with peripheral nerve stimulation. Oper Neurosurg. 2017;13(5):634–639. doi:10.1093/ons/opx017. PMID: 28922873.
3. Patil A, Otto D, Raikar S. Peripheral nerve field stimulation for sacroiliac joint pain. Neuromodulation. 2014;17(1):98–101. doi:10.1111/ner.12030

4. Chakrabortty S, Kumar S, Gupta D, Rudraraju S. Intractable sacroiliac joint pain treated with peripheral nerve field stimulation. J Anaesthesiol Clin Pharmacol. 2016;32(3):392–394. doi:10.4103/0970-9185.173336. PMID: 27625495; PMCID: PMC5009853.

5. Isu T, Kim K, Morimoto D, Iwamoto N. Superior and middle cluneal nerve entrapment as a cause of low back pain. Neurospine. 2018;15(1):25–32. doi:10.14245/ns.1836024.012. PMID: 29656623; PMCID: PMC5944640.

6. Tubbs RS, Levin MR, Loukas M, et al. Anatomy and landmarks for the superior and middle cluneal nerves: Application to posterior iliac crest harvest and entrapment syndromes. J Neurosurg Spine. 2010;13:356–359.

7. Konno T, Aota Y, Saito T, et al. Anatomical study of middle cluneal nerve entrapment. J Pain Res. 2017;10:1431–1435.

8. McGrath MC, Zhang M. Lateral branches of dorsal sacral nerve plexus and the long posterior sacroiliac ligament. Surg Radiol Anat. 2005;27:327–330.

9. Aota Y. Entrapment of middle cluneal nerves as an unknown cause of low back pain. World J Orthop. 2016;7:167–170.

10. Kim K, Isu T, Matsumoto J, et al. Low back pain due to middle cluneal nerve entrapment neuropathy. Eur Spine J. 2018;27(Suppl 3):309–313. https://doi.org/10.1007/s00586-017-5208-2

11. Murakami E, Tanaka Y, Aizawa T, et al. Effect of periarticular and intraarticular lidocaine injections for sacroiliac joint pain: Prospective comparative study. J Orthop Sci. 2007;12(3):274–280. doi:10.1007/s00776-007-1126-1. PMID: 17530380.

12. Fortin JD, Falco FJ. The Fortin finger test: An indicator of sacroiliac pain. Am J Orthop. 1997;26(7):477–480. PMID: 9247654.

13. Tunks ER, Crook J, Weir R. Epidemiology of chronic pain with psychological comorbidity: Prevalence, risk, course, and prognosis. Can J Psychiatry. 2008;53:224–234.

14. Evers AW, Kraaimaat FW, van Riel PL, Bijlsma JW. Cognitive, behavioral and physiological reactivity to pain as a predictor of long-term pain in rheumatoid arthritis patients. Pain. 2001;93:139–146.

15. Fishbain DA. Approaches to treatment decisions for psychiatric comorbidity in the management of the chronic pain patient. Med Clin North Am. 1999;83:737–760.

16. Jamison RN, Edwards RR, Liu X, et al. Relationship of negative affect and outcome of an opioid therapy trial among low back pain patients. Pain Pract. 2013;13(3):173–181.

17. Andersson HI, Ejlertsson G, Leden I, Schersten B. Impact of chronic pain on health care seeking, self-care, and medication. Results from a population-based Swedish study. J Epidemiol Commun Health. 1999;53:503–509.

18. Slavin KV. Peripheral nerve stimulation for neuropathic pain. Neurotherapeutics. 2008;5(1):100–106.

19. Narouze S, Benzon HT, Provenzano D, et al. Interventional spine and pain procedures in patients on antiplatelet and anticoagulant medications: Guidelines from the American Society of Regional Anesthesia and Pain Medicine, the European Society of Regional Anaesthesia and Pain Therapy, the American Academy of Pain Medicine, the International Neuromodulation Society, the North American Neuromodulation Society, and the World Institute of Pain. Reg Anesthes Pain Med. 2018;43:225–262.

20. Slavin KV. Peripheral nerve stimulation. Prog Neurol Surg. 2011;24:189–202.

21. Krishnan R, MacNeil SD, Malvankar-Mehta MS. Comparing sutures versus staples for skin closure after orthopaedic surgery: Systematic review and meta-analysis. BMJ Open. 2016;6(1):e009257.

22. Glennie RA, Korczak A, Naudie DD, et al. Monocryl and Dermabond vs staples in total hip arthroplasty performed through a lateral skin incision: A randomized controlled trial using a patient-centered assessment tool. J Arthroplasty. 2017;32(8):2431–2435.

23. Deer TR, Lamer TJ, Pope JE, et al. The Neurostimulation Appropriateness Consensus Committee (NACC) safety guidelines for the reduction of severe neurological injury. Neuromodulation. 2017;20(1):15–30. doi:10.1111/ner.12564. PMID: 28042918.

12

Preoperative considerations for peripheral nerve stimulation of the sacroiliac joint

Ajay B. Antony

Introduction

Careful attention to preoperative considerations for peripheral nerve stimulation (PNS) is paramount for optimizing patient safety and maximizing the effectiveness of the procedure to be performed. This involves considerations specific to the type of procedure being performed and minimizing patient risk factors that could lead to complications or poor outcomes. Preoperative planning begins in the exam room when the procedure is described to the patient and appropriate expectations are set. A description of risks, benefits, preoperative course, operative events, postoperative follow-up, and possible outcomes is the first step in ensuring good outcomes and a favorable risk/benefit profile.

This chapter reviews preoperative considerations for PNS of the sacroiliac joint (SIJ). It focuses on planning for the specific type of procedure being performed (trial vs. implant), risk stratification and patient optimization of underlying medical conditions, managing bleeding risk (anticoagulation), and minimizing risks of infection.

Preoperative evaluation

A thorough history and physical should be performed prior to any surgical procedure. This should be done at the time of initial identification of the patient as well as just before the procedure. Properly selected patients are those who have failed to find significant relief with conservative therapies, including physical therapy, oral analgesics, and simple injections. At the office visit, underlying patient comorbidities such as diabetes, cardiac disease, anticoagulation, and other health issues can be reviewed. Coordination with other physicians is sometimes necessary to address health concerns. Patient considerations related to the procedure itself may include factors that may make visualization with ultrasound or fluoroscopy difficult, such as prior surgery in the area or the patient's inability to assume the necessary position for the surgical procedure. A repeat evaluation must be performed just prior to the procedure to evaluate any changes in the patient's condition and to ensure that the patient carried out the preoperative directions (i.e., stopping anticoagulation).

Anesthesia

For either a trial or implant, the type of anesthesia to be administered must be considered. Many PNS procedures can be performed with local anesthesia only. Depending on physician and patient preference, sometimes a small amount of analgesic or anxiolytic medication can be administered through an intravenous line, providing conscious sedation. Especially when placing a lead in an area adjacent to or around a nerve, it is critical for the patient to be responsive to avoid unrecognized neural injury.

For an implant procedure, anesthetic techniques range from local only to moderate or deep sedation. General anesthesia can be considered under certain circumstances. In this case, an independent anesthesia provider is typically caring for the patient in an operating room setting. Before this, a proper preoperative evaluation for anesthesia use is necessary and should focus on cardiac risk stratification for non-cardiac surgery.

Anticoagulation management

Special consideration should be given to anticoagulation management when performing a PNS trial or implant. According to the 2018 American Society of Regional Anesthesiology guidelines, both a PNS trial and implant are considered low- to intermediate-risk procedures (Table 12.1). Peripheral neuromodulation is classified as a low- to intermediate-risk procedure, depending on the targeted nerve.[1] This depends on the specific location and invasiveness of the procedure. It is unlikely to encounter major vessels when using a posterior approach for PNS of the SIJ. Nevertheless, the proceduralist must have in-depth knowledge of the surrounding anatomy, including arterial and venous structures, to minimize this risk.

Table 12.2 summarizes the periprocedural management of anticoagulants and antiplatelet medications. A risk stratification must be done for each patient, weighing the potential for procedural bleeding against the cardiovascular risk of stopping the particular anticoagulant. Coordination with the specialist prescribing the anticoagulant is considered best practice.[1,2]

Risk of infection

Minimizing infectious risk begins with an evaluation of patient risk factors such as history of infection, diabetes, smoking, and hygiene. Any preexisting infections

TABLE 12.1 Pain procedures classified according to the potential risk of serious bleeding

High-risk procedures	Intermediate-risk procedures*	Low-risk procedures*
Spinal cord stimulation trial and implant	Interlaminar epidural steroid injections (cervical, thoracic, lumbar, sacral)	Peripheral nerve blocks
Dorsal root ganglion stimulation	Transforaminal epidural steroid injections (cervical, thoracic, lumbar, sacral)	Peripheral joint and musculoskeletal injections
Intrathecal catheter and pump implant		Trigger point injections, including piriformis injection
Vertebral augmentation (vertebroplasty and kyphoplasty)	Cervical** facet medial branch nerve blocks and radiofrequency ablation	Sacroiliac joint injections and sacral lateral branch blocks
Percutaneous decompression laminotomy	Intradiscal procedures (cervical, thoracic, lumbar)	Thoracic and lumbar facet medial branch nerve blocks and radiofrequency ablation
Epiduroscopy and epidural decompression	Sympathetic blocks (stellate, thoracic, splanchnic, celiac, lumbar, hypogastric)	PNS trial and implant***
	Trigeminal and sphenopalatine ganglia blocks	Pocket revision and implantable pulse generator/intrathecal pump replacement

*Patients with high risk of bleeding (old age, history of bleeding tendency, concurrent use of other anticoagulants/antiplatelets, liver cirrhosis or advanced liver disease, and advanced renal disease) undergoing low- or intermediate-risk procedures should be treated as intermediate or high risk, respectively.
**There is rich neck vascularity near target procedure site(s).
***Peripheral neuromodulation is low to intermediate risk, depending on the location of the target nerve in relation to critical vessels and the invasiveness of the procedure.

must be identified and treated. Modifiable risk factors should be addressed, such as lowering HbA1c and smoking cessation. For methicillin-resistant staphylococcus aureas (MRSA) carriers, 5 days of nasal mupirocin ointment is recommended for decolonization. Five days of chlorhexidine scrub is also recommended to minimize risk of infection.

All patients undergoing a PNS trial or implant should be managed with perioperative antibiotics. The selected agent should be determined prior to the day of surgery. In preparation for any trial or implant procedure, it is recommended to administer weight-based cefazolin within 1 hour of the incision. If the patient is allergic to or cannot tolerate cephalosporin, alternative antibiotics with broad coverage should be used. The routine use of vancomycin is not recommended.[3] Table 12.3 lists the infection-control measures recommended by the Centers for Disease Control and Prevention. The use of prophylactic antibiotic therapy is clinically supported by evidence-based studies.[3]

Conclusion

The preoperative evaluation and management of a patient undergoing PNS of the SIJ involves measures at several different phases of care. Optimization of patient comorbidities, appropriate management of anticoagulation, and planning strategies to minimize infection risk are paramount to ensure the best possible outcomes for the patient.

TABLE 12.2 Summary of periprocedural management of anticoagulants and antiplatelet medications

Drug	When to stop			When to restart
	High-risk procedures	Intermediate-risk procedures	Low-risk procedures	
ASA and ASA combinations	Primary prophylaxis: 6 d Secondary prophylaxis: shared assessment and risk stratification	Shared assessment and risk stratification*	No	24 h
Nonsteroidal anti-inflammatories (NSAIDs):	5 half-lives	No*	No	24 h
Diclofenac	1 d			
Ketorolac	1 d			
Ibuprofen	1 d			
Etodolac	2 d			
Indomethacin	2 d			
Naproxen	4 d			
Meloxicam	4 d			
Nabumetone	6 d			
Oxaprozin	10 d			
Piroxicam	10 d			
Phosphodiesterase inhibitors:				
Cilostazol	2 d	No	No	24 h
Dipyridamole	2 d	No	No	
ASA combinations	Follow ASA recommendations	Shared assessment and risk stratification		
Anticoagulants:			No, shared assessment and risk stratification	6 h
Coumadin	5 d, normal INR	5 d, normal INR		
Acenocoumarol	3 d, normal INR	3 d, normal INR	No, shared assessment and risk stratification	24 h
Intravenous heparin	6 h	6 h	6 h	2 h (if procedure was bloody, observe for 24 h)
Subcutaneous heparin, BID and TID	24 h	6 h	6 h	2 h (low-risk procedures); 6–8 h (intermediate-and high-risk procedures)
Low-molecular-weight heparin:				
Enoxaparin (prophylactic)	12 h	12 h	12 h	4 h (low-risk); 12–24 h (intermediate- and high-risk procedures)
Enoxaparin (therapeutic)	24 h	24 h	24 h	4 h (low-risk); 12–24 h (intermediate- and high-risk procedures)
Dalteparin	24 h	24 h	24 h	4 h (low-risk); 12–24 h (intermediate- and high-risk procedures)
Fibrinolytic agents	48 h	48 h	48 h	12 h if using normal daily dose once reinitiating 24 h if using loading dose once reinitiating
Fondaparinux	4 d	4 d	Shared assessment and risk stratification	6 h (low-risk); 24 h (intermediate- and high-risk procedures)

TABLE 12.2 Continued

Drug	When to stop			When to restart
	High-risk procedures	Intermediate-risk procedures	Low-risk procedures	
P2Y12 inhibitors:				
Clopidogrel	7 d	7 d	No, shared assessment and risk stratification	12–24 h
Prasugrel	7–10 d	7–10 d	No, shared assessment and risk stratification	24 h
Ticagrelor	5 d	5 d	No, shared assessment and risk stratification	24 h
Cangrelor	3 h	3 d	Shared assessment and risk stratification	24 h
New oral anticoagulants:				
Dabigatran	4 d, 4–6 d (impaired renal function)	4 d, 5–6 d (impaired renal function)	Shared assessment and risk stratification	24 h
Rivaroxaban	3 d	3 d	Shared assessment and risk stratification	24 h
Apixaban	3 d	3 d	Shared assessment and risk stratification	24 h
Edoxaban	3 d	3 d	Shared assessment and risk stratification	24 h
GP IIB/IIIa inhibitors:				
Abciximab	2–5 d	2–5 d	2–5 d	8–12 h
Eptifibatide	8–24 h	8–24 h	8–24 h	8–12 h
Tirofiban	8–24 h	8–24 h	8–24 h	8–12 h

* Specific anatomic configurations may increase the risk of procedural bleeding, such as interlaminar cervical epidural steroid injections.

TABLE 12.3 Infection-control measures recommended by the Centers for Disease Control and Prevention

Recommendations	Evidence rankings*
Preoperative measures:	
Optimize glucose control.	IB
Discontinue tobacco use.	IB
If hair is removed, use electric clippers immediately before surgery.	IA
Use prophylactic antibiotic therapy.	IA
Vancomycin should not be used routinely.	IB
Intraoperative measures:	
Use appropriate preparation technique and agent selection for skin antisepsis.	IB
Maintain positive pressure ventilation in the operating room (OR).	IB
Keep the OR doors closed during procedure.	IB
Limit OR traffic.	II
Handle tissue gently and eradicate dead space.	IB
Postoperative measures:	
Use occlusive sterile dressing for 4–48 hours postoperatively.	IB
If a dressing change is required, use:	
▪ Hand washing	IB
▪ Sterile technique	II

*CDC rankings: IA: Strongly recommended for implementation and supported by well-designed experimental, clinical, or epidemiological studies; IB: Strongly recommended for implementation and supported by some experimental, clinical, or epidemiological studies and strong theoretical rationale; II: Suggested for implementation and supported by suggestive clinical or epidemiological studies or theoretical rationale.

References

1. Deer TR, Narouze S, Provenzano DA, et al. The Neurostimulation Appropriateness Consensus Committee (NACC): Recommendations on bleeding and coagulation management in neurostimulation devices [published correction appears in Neuromodulation. 2017;20(4):407]. Neuromodulation. 2017;20(1):51–62. doi:10.1111/ner.12542

2. Narouze S, Benzon HT, Provenzano D, et al. Interventional spine and pain procedures in patients on antiplatelet and anticoagulant medications (second edition): Guidelines from the American Society of Regional Anesthesia and Pain Medicine, the European Society of Regional Anaesthesia and Pain Therapy, the American Academy of Pain Medicine, the International Neuromodulation Society, the North American Neuromodulation Society, and the World Institute of Pain. Reg Anesth Pain Med. 2018;43(3):225–262. doi: 10.1097/AAP.0000000000000700. PMID: 29278603.

3. Deer TR, Mekhail N, Provenzano D, et al. The appropriate use of neurostimulation of the spinal cord and peripheral nervous system for the treatment of chronic pain and ischemic diseases: The Neuromodulation Appropriateness Consensus Committee. Neuromodulation. 2014;17(6):515–550. doi:10.1111/ner.12208

13

Peripheral nerve stimulation trial and implantation

Kris Ferguson and Alaa Abd-Elsayed

Introduction

The nervous system is one of the most complex structures in the human body and is involved in many disease states. With neuropathic pain, the nervous system is intricately involved in the transduction, transmission, and perception of the disease state itself.[1-6]

Peripheral nerve stimulation (PNS) is the "direct electrical stimulation of identifiable and named nerves outside the neuroaxis, directly inhibiting primary afferents."[7] PNS has evolved from being a procedure that required careful, open dissection of the target nerve[8,9] to a sleek treatment requiring only image guidance and a minimally invasive percutaneous approach.[10,11] With the increased adoption of the percutaneous approach for PNS, the chronic pain industry has witnessed significant growth in the development of devices specifically for use in PNS procedures. This contrasts with the historical and off-label use of devices such as spinal cord stimulators implanted peripherally to treat neuralgia.

This chapter will detail the surgical recommendations and approaches to both successful trial stimulation and permanent implantation of PNS to treat sacroiliac joint (SIJ) pain. When using PNS to treat SIJ pain, the sacral dorsal rami of S1, S2, and S3 are the primary targets.[12] The SIJ is also innervated by the ventral rami of L4 and L5, the superior gluteal nerve, the dorsal rami of L5, and the middle cluneal nerve (Figure 13.1). The middle cluneal nerve is the sensory branch of the dorsal rami of S1, S2, and S3. It lies posterior to the posterior superior iliac spine to supply the posterior medial buttock area.[13] Typically, fluoroscopy is used for lead placement; however, ultrasound may be used to enhance lead placement.

History

PNS as a treatment for neuropathic pain originated in the 1960s. It is based on the gate-control theory for pain introduced by Melzack and Wall, who postulated that "innocuous

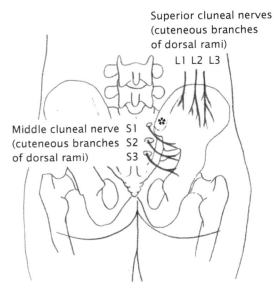

Superior cluneal nerves
(cuteneous branches
of dorsal rami)

L1 L2 L3

Middle cluneal nerve S1
(cuteneous branches S2
of dorsal rami) S3

FIGURE 13.1. Middle cluneal nerves of the SIJ. *Source:* From reference 24.

sensory information may suppress transmission of pain."[2] A 26-year-old woman with complex regional pain syndrome was the first documented person to have undergone a PNS surgery.

Unfortunately, PNS found little traction after its initial appearance in the 1960s. This was largely the result of a paucity of research related to these procedures and an overall lack of predictability and testability of the PNS approach itself. The overall result was a major obstacle to wide acceptance of the technique.

In the 1980s PNS started to gain legitimacy as an established surgical procedure. Weiner and Reed[4] pioneered various percutaneous techniques for electrode insertion in the vicinity of the occipital nerves for the treatment of occipital neuralgia. This was the start of the legitimacy of PNS for neuralgia. The significant observation was that an electric node in the vicinity of the nerve in question could achieve the same amount of pain relief as when the node is placed directly on the nerve. Thanks to Weiner and Reed, a less technically demanding and minimally invasive approach could be developed for the treatment of peripheral neuropathies.

Trial stimulation

A trial stimulation period that typically ranges from 7 to 14 days is standard in PNS as well as spinal cord stimulation.[14] The pain relief from the short-term PNS stimulation can persist even after the device has been removed. There are some newly developed devices that are never permanently implanted; rather, they are designed to be used for roughly 60 days and then removed, with results lasting for 12 or more months. The trial stimulation is an outpatient procedure in which temporary leads are placed and secured to the skin. These leads are attached to a temporary transmitter.[4] During the trial period patients record their pain daily. A trial stimulation is determined successful if it results in greater than 50% reduction in the patient's pain.[15] If greater than 50% pain relief is achieved, the patient may have the option to move forward with a permanent surgical implant. A failed stimulation trial is nearly always considered an absolute contraindication to permanent implantation as patients are extremely unlikely to benefit from the device.[14]

Trial stimulation procedure
Preparation

1. Obtain consent from the patient. Carefully describe the process and be sure to explain and carefully identify if any device is being used off-label. Ask the patient what questions they have.[14]
2. Prior to the procedure, evaluate and determine what the best anatomic position for the patient will be during the procedure.[16] Carefully determine what the best anatomic position will be for both the receiver and implantable lead associated with the device being used.
3. Position the patient for the procedure and use appropriate padding, as necessary.

Target point identification

1. Sterilely prepare and drape the affected area being supplied by the nerve[7] using institutional guidelines.
2. Determine the placement of the lead based on nerve stimulation and patient feedback.[7] The patient should report on stimulation intensity, location, and overall sensation.[4]
3. Lead placement can be performed using fluoroscopic or ultrasound guidance (or a combination of both) to identify the nerve and associated structures and/or landmarks.[10,11,14,17]
   a. If ultrasound is used, the physician will be able to visualize the nerve and adjacent structures.
   b. If fluoroscopy is used, a highly functional and working knowledge of the peripheral anatomy and the proper imaging modality is crucial to success.[18]
4. Identify the appropriate nerve(s) and/or landmark(s) for the trajectory path that has been defined for the stimulator lead placement.
5. Using a sterile marker, mark the skin at the point superficial to the target stimulation point (Figure 13.2).
6. Local anesthetic can be used to minimize procedure pain. Take care not to anesthetize the target nerve.
7. Use an introducer to create a channel for the trial lead placement (see Figure 13.3).

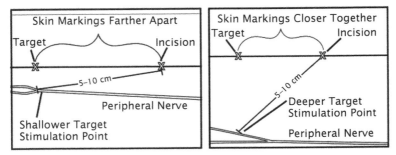

FIGURE 13.2. Skin markings and anticipated lead trajectory. *Source:* From reference 19.

    a. Some manufacturers use a "stimulation probe" designed to locate the target stimulation point for the lead placement.

    b. Some manufacturers may also provide a dilator, which can be used prior to the introducer (see Figure 13.3).

8. Once the introducer is in place, test for stimulation via the introducer needle.

    a. Some manufacturers require another type of lead or probe for this step.

9. Stimulation settings

    a. Verify that the output amplitude of the PNS device is set to zero.[19] Have your nonsterile assistant activate the device and slowly increase this amplitude until the patient reports discomfort or maximum output amplitude is reached (the maximum output amplitude will vary by PNS device).

    b. Tissue damage can occur if the PNS is set too high.

10. While the stimulation amplitude is in place, identify the location where paresthesia is produced in the sensory distribution of the target nerve.[19]

    a. Note the stimulation parameters identified by the patient, as these parameters may be useful if you intend to perform the permanent implantation at a later date.

    b. If paresthesia is not achieved, repositioning should be attempted. Do not bend the probe during this process.[19]

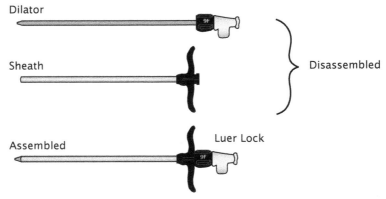

FIGURE 13.3. Introducer set. *Source:* From reference 19.

11. Identify the minimal stimulation needed to achieve paresthesia by decreasing the stimulation amplitude carefully by degrees.[19] When the paresthesia response is lost (as identified by the patient), slowly increase the stimulation until it is restored. Whatever the stimulation amplitude is upon the return of paresthesia is your minimum setting. Recommended minimum and maximum settings will be outlined by the device manufacturer and can vary by device.

12. Be cognizant of the depth and orientation of the probe, and take care to maintain it. Small movements can result in the loss of the identified location and can compromise your desired results (see Figure 13.4). Fluoroscopic imaging can be used to document your placement and can be referenced later when implanting a permanent lead.[18]

Lead insertion

1. With the introducer still in place, insert the device lead into the introducer (anchor end first if applicable). Individual devices have various ways of matching the introducer and lead systems (Figures 13.4, 13.5, and 13.6).

2. Firmly hold the lead in place in its position relative to the tissue.

3. Slowly retract the introducer to a predetermined manufacturer mark that allows for the stimulation end of the lead to be exposed below the skin entry site and thus allows for stimulation of the patient prior to full removal of the introducer itself.

4. Test the positioning of the stimulation lead by adjusting the amplitude as needed to produce anesthesia. Work with the patient to achieve desired effects. Record stimulation parameters for intraoperative use.

5. If the patient cannot identify the desired response, remove the introducer and lead together and inspect them for damage. If the components do not seem to have any damage, reinsert them and retry stimulation.

6. If the patient confirms proper lead placement, you can remove the introducer. Hold the lead and its loader (if applicable) in place. Slowly withdraw the introducer over the lead while applying (gentle) pressure to the tissue above and surrounding the stimulation end of the lead.[19] At this point, you should be left with the receiver end of the stimulation lead exiting through the skin and the simulation end of the lead in place underneath the skin.

7. Finally, connect the receiver end of the stimulation lead to the stimulation cable. The exact process and specifications for this step will vary by device and manufacturer.

8. Test for accurate placement of the lead using the PNS system.

   a. A patient response like the one that was previously documented should confirm placement.

   b. Some devices may have a predesigned system in place where the anchor is deployed in this step. If this is the case, there will be a predetermined place to withdraw the introducer, at which point the anchor will be deployed.

9. Per practitioner choice, you can use fluoroscopic imaging at this point to document anatomic positioning. This information can be used for future reference.

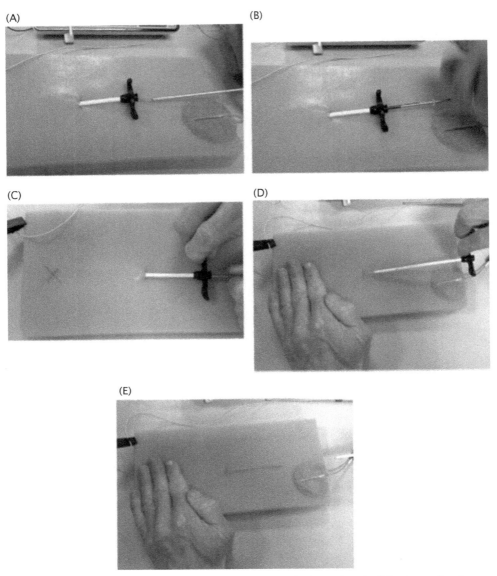

FIGURE 13.4. Lead deployment: (**A**) Insertion of introducer, (**B**) lead introduced, (**C**) lead retraction demonstrating lead contacts for testing, (**D**) anchor deployment, and (**E**) sheath removal. *Source:* From reference 7.

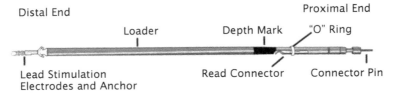

FIGURE 13.5. Sample lead. *Source:* From reference 19.

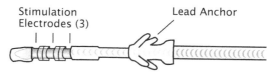

FIGURE 13.6. Sample lead stimulation end. *Source:* From reference 19.

10. The PNS system is secured with sterile dressing and bandages.
11. The leads are connected to a temporary transmitter/generator and secured to the patient.
12. The patient is sent home to record and evaluate the efficacy of the device on their chronic pain. Trial time depends on the device and whether it is a therapeutic or diagnostic PNS trial.

Permanent implantation only: tunneling and pocket dissection

The permanent implant procedure may or may not involve the implantation of an implantable pulse generator (IPG). Some PNS systems do not involve an IPG implant and instead rely on wireless technology. A generator is superficially placed in proximity to the implanted lead and secured by a band or specially designed clothing. The generator overlying the lead supplies the power necessary to provide stimulation. For the implanted IPG, the permanent implant procedure is similar to the trial procedure, with the addition of tunneling the receiver end of the lead through the subcutaneous tissue to connect it to the IPG, which will also be implanted in a predetermined site in the body.

1. Follow the steps previously outlined for preparation, target point identification, and lead insertion. Use the imaging and amplitude settings you previously recorded.
2. Once successful stimulation is determined, secure the ends of the stimulating electrode to the underlying fascia (the manufacturer will often provide an anchor or fastener for this purpose).
3. At this time, it is typical for the patient to receive a short-acting anesthetic for use during the tunneling process.
4. The receiver end of the leads should not cross any joint lines and must terminate in an area of the patient's body where they can tolerate it.
5. Identify and mark the insertion site for the tunneling needle.[19] The tunneling needle should be inserted where you anticipate the receiver end of the lead to terminate (see Figures 13.7, 13.8, and 13.9).

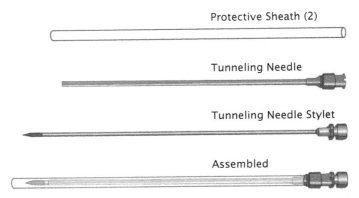

FIGURE 13.7. Tunneling needle and tunneling needle stylet components and assembly. *Source:* From reference 19.

Tunneling needles are very sharp; proceed with caution.

6. Local anesthetic should be injected subcutaneously along the anticipated tunneling tract.
7. Make a stab incision that reaches through the subcutaneous layer for the tunneling needle insertion point.[19]
8. Insert the tunneling needle as parallel as possible to the skin's surface (see Figure 13.9).
9. Keep the tunneling needle as superficial/shallow as possible while you tunnel from the tunneling insertion site underneath the skin to the incision site (target nerve).
10. Once you arrive at the incision site and are positioned next to the receiving end of the lead, remove the tunneling needle stylet, which will leave only the needle in place (see Figures 13.7 and 13.9).
11. Carefully insert the receiver end of the stimulation lead into the distal end of the tunneling needle. Make sure there is no slack in the lead (see Figure 13.8). Take care not to pinch or damage the lead during this process.[19] If you must use forceps, work to avoid those with teeth.
12. Once the receiver end of the lead has been successfully threaded through the tunneling needle, apply pressure to the tissue at the incision site to prevent lead migration while you withdraw the tunneling needle (see Figure 13.10).

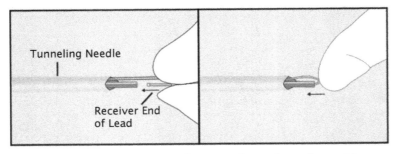

FIGURE 13.8. Tunneling needle with receiver end insertion. *Source:* From reference 19.

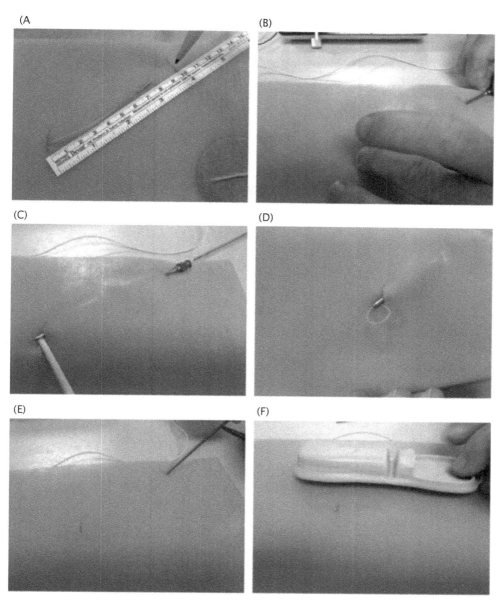

FIGURE 13.9. Finalizing lead placement: (**A**) Measurement of lead and second incision site, (**B, C**) placement of the tunneling device, (**D**) lead placement within the tunneler, (**E**) tunneler removal, and (**F**) final lead placement. In the device demonstrated here, there is no pocket dissection as the device has an overlying external pulse generator. *Source:* From reference 7.

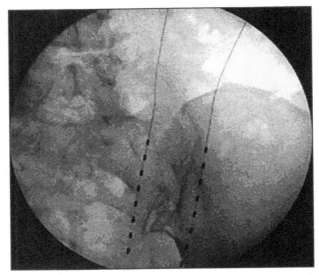

FIGURE 13.10. Image of leads targeting the sacral lateral branches. *Source:* From reference 12.

13. Initiate pocket dissection as necessary based on the device. Be sure to use a topical anesthetic during this process, and be sure to stay above the fascia. The pocket should be just large enough to insert the IPG part of the device into (see Figure 13.11).

14. It is advisable to use fluoroscopic imaging to document the placement of the receiver end of the lead and the IPG.

15. Use standard wound-closure techniques to close the pocket. Sutures are typically used.

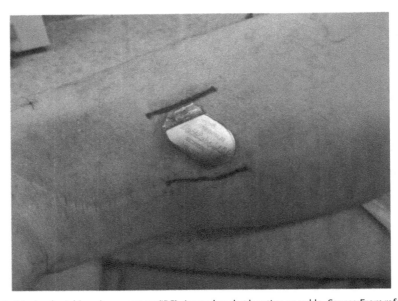

FIGURE 13.11. Implantable pulse generator (IPG) size and pocket location on ankle. *Source:* From reference 25.

16. Advise the patient regarding signs of potential infection or irritation: newly developed erythema, induration, or pain, which may or may not be expanding; new-onset fever or general feelings of malaise). Follow-up visits will vary depending on individual patient and device needs.

Conclusion

The slow uptake of PNS as a viable therapy for chronic pain was due to the cumbersome initial surgical approaches. PNS placement used to require the careful dissection of a nerve with a multi-contact electrode (paddle) placed longitudinally or immediately adjacent to the nerve itself.[20] This open approach could lead to serious complications, most of them iatrogenic.[21,22] Nerve injury was common and revision rates exceeded 85%.[23]

Everything changed with the development of the percutaneous approach for PNS placement in 1999.[4] This approach allowed for a much more efficient surgical process with the same or increased efficacy. Complications were significantly reduced, and the types of complications were significantly less morbid. The improved efficacy and decreased complication rate invited the much-needed investment and interest of device manufacturers, who took on the task of acquiring approval from the Food and Drug Administration (FDA) via device trials.

Understanding the percutaneous approach from a surgical process standpoint is essential for any chronic pain practitioner. The purpose of this chapter was to outline, step by step, the overarching implantation process for newly developed PNS devices that solely use the percutaneous approach.

References

1. Slavin, K. V. In *Peripheral nerve stimulation* (Vol. 24, pp. 1–15; Karger Publishers, 2011).
2. Melzack, R., & Wall, P. D. Pain mechanisms: A new theory. *Science* **150**, 971–979, doi:10.1126/science.150.3699.971 (1965).
3. Sweet, W. H. Control of pain by direct electrical stimulation of peripheral nerves. *Clin Neurosurg* **23**, 103–111, doi:10.1093/neurosurgery/23.cn_suppl_1.103 (1976).
4. Weiner, R. L., & Reed, K. L. Peripheral neurostimulation for control of intractable occipital neuralgia. *Neuromodulation* **2**, 217–221 (1999).
5. Yamanaka, H., & Noguchi, K. Pathophysiology of neuropathic pain: Molecular mechanisms underlying central sensitization in the dorsal horn in neuropathic pain. *Brain Nerve* **64**, 1255–1265 (2012).
6. Liu, F., & Yuan, H. Role of glia in neuropathic pain. *Front Biosci* **19**, 798–807 (2014).
7. Deer, T. R., Pope, J. E., & Kaplan, M. A novel method of neurostimulation of the peripheral nervous system: The StimRouter implantable device. *Tech Reg Anesth Pain Manag* **16**, 113–117 (2012).
8. Hassenbusch, S. J., Stanton-Hicks, M., Schoppa, D., et al. Long-term results of peripheral nerve stimulation for reflex sympathetic dystrophy. *J Neurosurg* **84**, 415–423 (1996).
9. Stanton-Hicks, M., & Salamon, J. Stimulation of the central and peripheral nervous system for the control of pain. *J Clin Neurophysiol* **14**, 46–62 (1997).
10. Huntoon, M. A., Huntoon, E. A., Obray, J. B., & Lamer, T. J. Feasibility of ultrasound-guided percutaneous placement of peripheral nerve stimulation electrodes in a cadaver model: Part one, lower extremity. *Reg Anesth Pain Med* **33**, 551–557 (2008).

11. Huntoon, M. A., Hoelzer, B. C., Burgher, A. H., et al. Feasibility of ultrasound-guided percutaneous placement of peripheral nerve stimulation electrodes and anchoring during simulated movement: Part two, upper extremity. *Reg Anesth Pain Med* **33**, 558–565 (2008).

12. Chakrabortty, S., Kumar, S., Gupta, D., & Rudraraju, S. Intractable sacroiliac joint pain treated with peripheral nerve field stimulation. *J Anaesthesiol Clin Pharmacol* **32**(3), 392–394 (2016).

13. Konno, T., Aota, Y., Saito, T., et al. Anatomical study of middle cluneal nerve entrapment. *J Pain Res* **10**, 1431–1435 (2017).

14. Slavin, K. V. History of peripheral nerve stimulation. *Prog Neurol Surg* **24**, 1–15, 2011, doi:10.1159/000323002.

15. Becser, N., Bovim, G., & Sjaastad, O. Extracranial nerves in the posterior part of the head: Anatomic variations and their possible clinical significance. *Spine* **23**, 1435–1441 (1998).

16. Gilmore, C. A., Kapural, L., McGee, M. J., & Boggs, J. W. Percutaneous peripheral nerve stimulation for chronic low back pain: Prospective case series with 1 year of sustained relief following short-term implant. *Pain Practice* **20**, 310–320 (2020).

17. Huntoon, M. A., & Burgher, A. H. Ultrasound-guided permanent implantation of peripheral nerve stimulation (PNS) system for neuropathic pain of the extremities: Original cases and outcomes. *Pain Med* **10**, 1369–1377 (2009).

18. Loukas, M., El-Sedfy, A., Tubbs, R. S., et al. Identification of greater occipital nerve landmarks for the treatment of occipital neuralgia. *Folia Morphologica* **65**, 337–342 (2006).

19. Bioness. StimRouter Neuromodulation System. (2019).

20. Mobbs, R., Nair, S., & Blum, P. Peripheral nerve stimulation for the treatment of chronic pain. *J Clin Neurosci* **14**, 216–221 (2007).

21. Nielson, K., Watts, C., & Clark, W. Peripheral nerve injury from implantation of chronic stimulating electrodes for pain control. *Surg Neurol* **5**, 51–53 (1976).

22. Kirsch, W., Lewis, J., & Simon, R. Experiences with electrical stimulation devices for the control of chronic pain. *Med Instrum* **9**, 217–220 (1975).

23. Nashold Jr, B., Goldner, J., Mullen, J., & Bright, D. Long-term pain control by direct peripheral-nerve stimulation. *J Bone Joint Surg* **64**, 1–10 (1982).

24. Sittitavornwong, S., Falconer, D. S., Shah, R., et al. Anatomic considerations for posterior iliac crest bone procurement. *J Oral Maxillofac Surg* **71**, 1777–1788 (2013).

25. Reverberi, C., Dario, A., Barolat, G., & Zuccon, G. Using peripheral nerve stimulation (PNS) to treat neuropathic pain: A clinical series. *Neuromodulation* **17**, 777–783 (2014).

14

Outcome measures and outcomes of peripheral nerve stimulation of the sacroiliac joint

Hunter Hoopes and Mayank Gupta

Introduction

The measurement of pain has proven to be difficult for pain management clinicians and researchers alike. Pain is an abstract and subjective sensation that differs widely between patients. Further complicating the ability to measure pain is the idea that the perception of pain is multifactorial, stemming from a combination of somatic dysfunctions as well as psychological stressors. The challenge is being able to translate this complex and subjective perception of pain into an objective data point that can be measured over time. Due to the complexity of the perception of pain, assessing outcomes after pain management interventions can be challenging.

To be effective, outcome measures of pain need to be valid, reproducible, and applicable for a wide range of patients. Several different outcome measures exist, and each demonstrates its own utility. However, the ability to use these scaling systems often depends on how easily it can be administered and how well patients can understand what is being asked of them. Often the precision and validity of certain pain scoring systems are sacrificed for quicker and easier-to-administer scales. Because several different pain assessment scales have been developed, with extensive variability between them, Dworkin et al.[1] in 2003 published recommendations of outcome measures, known as the Initiative on Methods, Measurements, and Pain Assessment in Clinical Trials (IMMPACT), to review which measures were the most appropriate to use in measuring the following domains:

- Pain
- Physical functioning

- Emotional functioning
- Participant ratings of global improvement and satisfaction with treatment
- Symptoms and adverse events
- Participant disposition

In this chapter we review some of the more common outcome measures that have been recommended to be used both clinically and in research to measure chronic pain. We also discuss the outcome measures that have been used specifically in the setting of peripheral nerve stimulation (PNS) of the sacroiliac joint (SIJ) and which pain scoring systems could be used in the future to improve our understanding of the patient's perception of pain improvement with neuromodulation of the SIJ.

Visual analog scale and numeric rating scale

The visual analog scale (VAS), a commonly used measure of pain, consists of a line that is usually 10 cm long and is anchored by two verbal descriptors of pain, each representing an extreme (Figure 14.1).[2,3] A zero on the VAS represents no pain at all; a 10 represents the worst pain imaginable. Respondents mark a line on the scale that they feel represents their pain at that moment.[2] The numeric rating scale (NRS) is very similar to the VAS. It consists of an 11-point scaling system (0–10) with the extremes of the scale similar to the VAS, but it can be administered completely verbally.[2]

The VAS and NRS provide a representation of pain only at a single point of time and provide no insight into the quality of the pain. However, what the VAS and NRS lack in data, they make up for in ease of administration: They can be administered in less than a minute and require no prior training.[2] This makes these pain scale measures some of the most commonly used because they can be administered by clinic staff and can be asked about quickly at each follow-up visit. Furthermore, while these scales might differ greatly between patients, high test–retest reliability has been shown with these assessments,[2] making them useful to track a patient's pain over time.

Pain medication dependence

One objective measure of the success of an intervention is the patient's dependence on oral pain medications after the procedure. Especially in the setting of an opioid epidemic, one goal of interventional pain management is to decrease the dependence on oral medications.

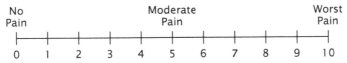

FIGURE 14.1. Representation of the VAS.[3] Patients are easily able to stratify their level of pain by indicating with a pencil where their pain falls along the spectrum.

Questions about the quantity of medications and how long the patient can last before requiring rescue analgesics are essential to provide insight into a patient's level of pain.[1] With electronic medical records, medication requirements can easily be tracked over time and can be used to assess the long-term efficacy of pain interventions. In research settings, this outcome measure can also facilitate inclusion of a placebo group because, in theory, a placebo group would require more dependence on oral analgesics than an experimental group that underwent a form of true intervention.[1]

West Haven-Yale Multidimensional Pain Inventory Interference Scale

While the VAS and NRS are lauded for their simplicity, at the other end of the spectrum exists the West Haven-Yale Multidimensional Pain Inventory Interference Scale (WHYMPI). The WHYMPI is a much more comprehensive questionnaire that, rather than assigning a simple numeric value to the pain, was designed to evaluate chronic pain from a cognitive-behavioral perspective and assess the level of physical function of patients despite their pain.[1,4]

The WHYMPI consists of three sections. The first section asks patients to respond on a seven-point scale (0–6) regarding six general concepts: pain severity, interference of pain in their life, dissatisfaction of the effect of their pain on functional ability, evaluation of familial support, perceived life control, and distress in their life caused by the pain.[4] The second section was designed to evaluate patients' perceptions of their significant other's reaction to their pain, such as how helpful the significant other is with their pain, how often they are ignored by their significant other, or how often the significant other expresses irritation or frustration with the patient because of their pain.[4] The final section indicates how often the patient is able to engage in predetermined common activities such as washing dishes, grocery shopping, and preparing a meal, among other items.[4]

One of the several benefits of this questionnaire is that it can be applied to any form of chronic pain. The WHYMPI not only shows the limitations that the patient's pain causes in their life but also the way that they cope with the pain and the support they have to deal with the pain.[5] It has also been shown to have high test–retest stability, which makes it a useful tool for measuring chronic pain.[5] However, due to the complexity of the test and the time it takes for a patient to complete the test, the WHYMPI seems to have more utility to establish a baseline for the patient. Because of the length of the questionnaire, patients may often need assistance or may refuse to complete it at each follow-up visit in the clinic, which decreases the practicality of the WHYMPI.

Brief Pain Inventory

The Brief Pain Inventory (BPI) is recommended as a method for assessing physical function in patients with chronic pain based on IMMPACT recommendations.[1] There are two forms, the short form and long form; the short form is more widely used. The goal of the BPI is similar to the WHYMPI except it is considerably simpler than the WHYMPI. The BPI and short-form BPI consist of a questionnaire that can be self-administered since the questions and scoring are easy to understand. It takes into account the patient's pain at its worse, the best, and the average pain level they experience on a normal day. It then asks about the interference that their pain causes in their daily life, such as the effect on their walking, mood, relationships, sleep, and life enjoyment, among other items.[6,7,8]

Because of the simplicity of the BPI, it can be used in a clinical setting without placing a burden on clinical staff. Although it was originally developed to measure pain and functional ability in cancer patients, it has been shown in the literature to have similar validity in patients with other forms of chronic pain.[6] It has also been shown to be sensitive to changes in pain over time, making it a reliable follow-up tool in the clinic.[6]

Oswestry Disability Index

The Oswestry Disability Index (ODI) is one of the most widely recommended outcome measures for chronic pain from spinal disorders.[9] It is quick to complete and easy for patients to understand, and it provides a quantitative measure in the form of a percentage to measure the disability that the pain is causing to the patient.[9]

The ODI questionnaire requests that patients circle a statement that best describes them in 10 different domains: pain intensity, personal care, lifting, walking, sitting, standing, sleeping, sex life, social life, and traveling.[9] Each domain contains six statements representing the spectrum of disability that the pain causes.[9] The statement of least severity is scored as a 0, and the most severe is 5, for a maximum of 50 points. To score a questionnaire, the patient's responses are graded and divided by 50 total points and multiplied by 100 to create a percentage.[9] For instance, a patient's response score of 20 is divided by 50, then multiplied by 100, resulting in an ODI of 40%.

The ease of the ODI and the comprehensive lifestyle factors that it measures create a reliable outcome measure of physical function. While certainly not perfect, it seems to be a reliable outcome measure for clinical or research use. It can be easily trended over time to demonstrate the effectiveness of interventional procedures. Box 14.1 shows the ODI version 2.1a.

Beck Depression Inventory

While treating the patient's somatic complaints, it is important not to forget the effect that chronic pain can have on psychological health. By some estimates, as many as 85% of patients with chronic pain also struggle with depression.[10] Occasionally the pain directly contributes to the development of depression, but sometimes the opposite is true and depression can lead to chronic pain.[10] Therefore, equally as important as measuring pain scores in response to treatment is measuring emotional functioning. The Beck Depression Inventory (BDI) is a questionnaire that assigns a score of 0 to 3 (on a 4-point scale) for 21 different questions designed to assess the level of depression a patient may be experiencing.[11] It is scored by

BOX 14.1. Example of the ODI questionnaire. Used with permission

Section 1 - Pain intensity
- ○ I have no pain at the moment.
- ○ The pain is very mild at the moment.
- ○ The pain is moderate at the moment.
- ○ The pain is fairly severe at the moment.
- ○ The pain is very severe at the moment.
- ○ The pain is the worst imaginable at the moment.

Section 2 - Personal care (washing, dressing, etc.)
- ○ I can look after myself normally without causing additional pain.
- ○ I can look after myself normally but it is very painful.
- ○ It is painful to look after myself and I am slow and careful.
- ○ I need some help but manage most of my personal care.
- ○ I need help every day in most aspects of my personal care.
- ○ I do not get dressed, I wash with difficulty and stay in bed.

Section 3 - Lifting
- ○ I can lift heavy weights without additional pain.
- ○ I can lift heavy weights but it gives me additional pain.
- ○ Pain prevents me from lifting heavy weights off the floor but I can manage if they are conveniently positioned, e.g. on a table.
- ○ Pain prevents me from lifting heavy weights but I can manage light to medium weights if they are conveniently positioned.
- ○ I can only lift very light weights.
- ○ I cannot lift or carry anything at all.

Section 4 - Walking
- ○ Pain does not prevent me from walking any distance.
- ○ Pain prevents me from walking more than one mile.
- ○ Pain prevents me from walking more than a quarter of a mile.
- ○ Pain prevents me from walking more than 100 yards.
- ○ I can only walk using a cane or crutches.
- ○ I am in bed most of the time and have to crawl to the toilet.

Section 5 - Sitting

- O I can sit in any chair as long as I like.
- O I can sit in my favorite chair as long as I like.
- O Pain prevents me from sitting for more than 1 hour.
- O Pain prevents me from sitting for more than half an hour.
- O Pain prevents me from sitting for more than 10 minutes.
- O Pain prevents me from sitting at all.

Section 6 - Standing

- O I can stand as long as I want without additional pain.
- O I can stand as long as I want but it gives me additional pain.
- O Pain prevents me from standing for more than 1 hour.
- O Pain prevents me from standing for more than half an hour.
- O Pain prevents me from standing for more than 10 minutes.
- O Pain prevents me from standing at all.

Section 7 - Sleeping

- O My sleep is never interrupted by pain.
- O My sleep is occasionally interrupted by pain.
- O Because of pain I have less than 6 hours sleep.
- O Because of pain I have less than 4 hours sleep.
- O Because of pain I have less than 2 hours sleep.
- O Pain prevents me from sleeping at all.

Section 8 - Sex life (if applicable)

- O My sex life is normal and causes no additional pain.
- O My sex life is normal but causes some additional pain.
- O My sex life is nearly normal but is very painful.
- O My sex life is severely restricted by pain.
- O My sex life is nearly non existent because of pain.
- O Pain prevents me from having any sex life at all.

Section 9 - Social life

- O My social life is normal and causes me no additional pain.
- O My social life is normal but increases the degree of pain.
- O Pain has no significant effect on my social life apart from limiting my more energetic interests, e.g. sport, etc.
- O Pain has restricted my social life and I do not go out as often.
- O Pain has restricted my social life to home.
- O I have no social life because of pain.

Section 10 - Traveling
- ○ I can travel anywhere without pain.
- ○ I can travel anywhere but it gives me additional pain.
- ○ Pain is bad but I am able to manage trips over two hours.
- ○ Pain restricts me to trips of less than one hour.
- ○ Pain restricts me to short necessary trips of under 30 minutes.
- ○ Pain prevents me from traveling except to receive treatment.

Result
Your ODI = ☐ %
ODI © Jeremy Fairbank, 1980. All Rights Reserved.
ODI - United States/English - Version of 29 Jul 11 - Mapi Institute.

adding up each of the responses and stratifies patients into groups of either normal, mild mood disturbance, borderline clinical depression, moderate depression, severe depression, or extreme depression.[11]

The BDI is a quick screening tool that can be used to assess a patient's emotional function in response to pain and help identify which patients would benefit from further psychological counseling and therapy as an adjunct to their pain treatment. Even after treating somatic complaints, a patient suffering from psychological distress may not report benefit from the intervention, which is why the BDI is an outcome measure that should be used in patients with chronic pain.

Patient Global Impression of Change scale

Self-reported improvement in pain remains the gold standard of measuring outcomes.[1] The Patient Global Impression of Change (PGIC) scale is a simple single question of how much patients feel that they have improved, graded on a 7-point scale ranging from very much worse (7), to no change (4), with very much improved (1) being at the positive end of the spectrum.[1] This simple question allows practitioners to measure the improvement of all interventions since a patient began care at the clinic and is an important indicator of overall patient satisfaction. Box 14.2 provides an example of the PGIC.

Adverse events and complications

Every intervention in medicine has the potential to do harm, and one outcome that is essential to measure regardless of the treatment is adverse events and complications. Depending on the intervention, complications or adverse events can range from benign to life threatening, and measurement of these events is important in determining a treatment's efficacy.

Adverse events and complications can be measured in several ways. The most common methods include questionnaires and checklists for the patient to complete. However, when checklists are used, adverse events are more likely to be reported,[12] possibly because of recall bias. Sometimes adverse effects are listed in consent forms, which may lead to patients opting not to be treated[12] or may make patients more aware of potential side effects that they might otherwise not notice. These pitfalls make measurement of adverse events more complicated.

At the very least, interviewing patients using open-ended questions allows assessment of adverse events that are clinically significant and that patients have noticed affecting their day-to-day life.[1] It is also important to evaluate the severity of the complications. For example, two studies may have a similar incidence of adverse effects but a dramatically different severity of complications,[12] demonstrating why severity is a crucial portion of this outcome measure.

Participant disposition

The IMMPACT recommendations discuss participant disposition as another core outcome measure in the setting of clinical trials. Dworkin et al.[1] suggest that valuable information to report includes the recruitment process, the number of candidates who were excluded and why, the number of candidates who chose not to participate and why, the use of prohibited concomitant medications, the number of subjects who did not complete the study and why, and the reasons and types of nonadherence to the treatment protocol. When reported, this information provides insight into the true efficacy and applicability of the data, and whether or not the results will be able to be replicated in a clinical setting. Poorly designed studies may create unrealistic situations: While the data may appear promising, the findings may not have similar outcomes in the real world.

BOX 14.2. Example of the PGI-C

PATIENT GLOBAL IMPRESSION OF CHANGE (PGIC)

Since the start of the study, my overall status is:
✓*one box only:*

[1] ☐ Very Much Improved
[2] ☐ Much Improved
[3] ☐ Minimally Improved
[4] ☐ No Change
[5] ☐ Minimally Worse
[6] ☐ Much Worse
[7] ☐ Very Much Worse

(US /English)

Zurich Claudication Questionnaire

While the previously mentioned outcome measures are recommended as core outcome measures for clinical trials on chronic pain per the IMMPACT recommendations, some other outcome measures specific to certain forms of chronic pain are worth discussing. In 2014, the MiDAS ENCORE study looked at the outcomes with the minimally invasive lumbar decompression procedure or epidural steroid injections in patients with lumbar spinal stenosis and claudication symptoms. As the primary outcome measure, the researchers used the ODI, and secondary measures included the NRS pain scale and the Zurich Claudication Questionnaire (ZCQ).[13] The ZCQ was also an outcome measure in a 2008 clinical trial investigating the efficacy of the Vertiflex Superion Interspinous Spacer.[14]

The ZCQ, developed in 1995, evaluates the physical limitations and symptoms of patients with spinal stenosis.[15,16] It consists of two scales, the first measuring the severity of patient symptoms and the second focused on functional limitations. It is a comprehensive questionnaire that evaluates the pain, balance deficits, and neuroischemic symptoms associated with lumbar spinal stenosis.[15,16] It has been found to have high accuracy and reliability in measuring the functional ability of patients with lumbar spinal stenosis, making it an effective outcome measure to consider when evaluating patients who present with lower back pain.[15,16]

Western Ontario and McMaster Universities Osteoarthritis Index

Osteoarthritis is a common cause of chronic pain. The Western Ontario and McMaster Universities Osteoarthritis index (WOMAC) is a scale that was originally developed to measure functional disability of patients with hip and knee osteoarthritis and was intended to measure improvement in response to treatment. However, studies suggest that it also has reliability when applied to other joints with osteoarthritis.[17]

The WOMAC scale evaluates three domains related to osteoarthritis: pain, stiffness, and functional assessment.[17] The pain domain asks patients to address pain severity in five different scenarios and to rate their pain on a scale of 0 to 4. The second domain addresses stiffness severity in the joint in the morning and in the evening on a scale of 0 to 4, and the final domain asks patients to rate their difficulty with 17 different actions on a scale of 0 to 4.[18] Scores from each section are then added together to produce a final score,[18] which can be followed to show improvement after treatment. It has been shown to have high test–retest reliability, validity, and responsiveness[17] to change, making it an excellent measure to evaluate patients with osteoarthritis.

Outcome measures used for PNS of the SIJ

SIJ dysfunction is a common cause of chronic lower back pain and is estimated to be prevalent in 10% to 30% of patients who present with lower back pain.[19] Diagnosis of SIJ pathology can be difficult because diagnostic SIJ injections can yield a 20% false-positive rate.[19] This makes it clinically very difficult to distinguish from other causes of lower back pain. Even after a correct diagnosis is made, treatment can often be difficult due to the incredible anatomic variability between articular surfaces and a complicated network of nerves innervating the SIJ.[20] Peripheral neuromodulation has been demonstrated to be one of the effective options for the treatment of SIJ dysfunction.

Like any procedure, the outcome of PNS for the SIJ depends on appropriate patient selection. Comorbidities such as obesity, which could affect lead placement,[21] or psychological evaluations to rule out somatization or untreated depression,[22] are important factors to consider when identifying which patients could benefit from neuromodulation. Although diagnostic SIJ injections have low specificity, there is moderate evidence to support the use of diagnostic SIJ injections to demonstrate that the patient's pain is originating from the SIJ.[19] Greater than 50% improvement in pain with a trial of stimulation can also be used to predict success with long-term PNS.[23]

As mentioned previously, translating the perception of pain into a data point can prove challenging because pain perception is subjective and varies so widely between patients. The most common scaling systems identified in the literature to measure outcomes of neuromodulation have been the VAS pain score and ODI, although other measures include a decrease in pain medications and overall patient satisfaction. In June 2012, the SENZA-RCT clinical trial aimed to demonstrate the noninferiority of the Senza spinal cord stimulator to other commercially available spinal cord stimulators. The outcome measures that the researchers used to demonstrate this were primarily the change in VAS pain score, the ODI, and the number of subjects with adverse events.[24]

The data supporting the effectiveness of PNS has been largely collected through retrospective and prospective cohort studies. In 2018 Goroszeniuk[20] conducted a retrospective review of a cohort of 12 patients who underwent PNS for the SIJ between 18 to 36 months and demonstrated a decrease in the VAS pain score from 8.7 ± 1.1 preoperatively to 1.1 ± 1.0 ($p = .001$). The patients also reported that the impact of pain on their daily life decreased from $94.1 \pm 5.9\%$ to $5.8 \pm 6.0\%$ ($p = .001$) averaged over several assessments within 16 months of the implant. Overall patient satisfaction after the procedure among this cohort ranged from 80% to 100%. A prospective cohort study in 2017 by Guentchev et al.[23] followed 16 patients with refractory SIJ pain. Two months after implantation, the patients' mean VAS score decreased from 8.8 to 1.3 and the ODI decreased from 58% to 13%. At 6 months the average ODI was 23% ($p = .0006$) and VAS score was 1.9 ($p < .001$).

In a 2014 retrospective cohort study of 10 patients, Patil et al.[22] demonstrated that six out of 10 patients treated with PNS for the SIJ were able to reduce their medication regimens, and four out of 10 reported improvement of their sleep patterns. Six out of 10 also reported a decrease in 50% or more in their VAS pain score. In 2015 Guentchev et al.[25] demonstrated that eight out of 11 patients treated decreased their pain medication regimen by at least 50% postoperatively.

Studies into the effectiveness of PNS for the SIJ are limited due to the small cohorts in each study. Additionally, published data cannot account for possible differences that may exist between manufacturers of PNS equipment, such as Medtronic, St. Jude, or Boston

Scientific. Furthermore, due to ethical limitations, PNS devices were not able to be turned off to conduct double-blinded studies. Interestingly, in the previously mentioned cohort study by Guentchev et al.,[23] six patients unknowingly experienced an interruption in stimulation due to accidental deactivation or end of battery life. All six of these patients promptly experienced return of their pain, and the researchers concluded that this supports the notion that their pain relief was not due to the placebo effect.

In small cohorts, PNS for chronic SIJ pain has been shown to decrease pain scores, increase functionality, and decrease dependence on oral pain medications. Although there are no large double-blinded clinical trials that demonstrate the effectiveness of neuromodulation for the SI joint, initial data from small cohorts suggest that it will be a valuable tool in treating these patients and at least warrants consideration when treating patients with intractable SIJ pain.

A review of the literature of neuromodulation for the SIJ mainly yielded retrospective cohort studies and case studies. Because of this, some outcome measures were not able to be evaluated. In future larger-scale studies of neuromodulation of the SIJ, one important outcome measure that should also be identified is the BDI. This recommendation stems from the idea that many patients with SIJ pain are misdiagnosed as having lower back pain and have often undergone several treatments over several years with no improvement. As stated previously, psychological distress is associated with chronic pain, and many patients express feelings of hopelessness as they undergo treatment after treatment with no relief. Therefore, evaluation of the BDI allows practitioners to establish a baseline of patients' psychological well-being and follow their psychological improvement in response to treatment.

Another important outcome measure that should continue to be measured in future studies into the effectiveness of neuromodulation of the SIJ is the patient's dependence on pain medications. Of the literature available for neuromodulation of the SIJ, only two cohort studies measured oral medication requirements. In the face of an opioid epidemic, medical professionals are increasingly being encouraged to move away from oral opioid medications if possible, and neuromodulation appears to be a promising modality to accomplish this. Demonstration of decreased opioid requirements in future PNS studies could promote more widespread use of this modality and increase patient awareness of neuromodulation as an option for chronic pain.

Conclusion

Determining which outcome measure to use depends on what parameters the clinician wants to measure. Scaling systems should be easy to administer while still providing the level of detail required to understand the patient's pain. Simple numeric values of pain, such as the NRS and VAS, are quick and easy to use, which is why they are among the most commonly used outcome measures despite the small amount of information they assess. However, despite this they provide a relatively reliable value to measure a patient's pain over time. The ODI and BPI offer more insight into the functional limitations that patients may have because of their pain and also offer high test–retest reliability and relative ease of administration. Psychological evaluation using outcome measures such as the BDI is important for measuring the psychological aspect that pain has on a patient's life. Clinicians should remember to identify this, as pain is a subjective psychological sensation of a somatic dysfunction. The most common of these outcomes used in the literature to measure the impact of neuromodulation of the SIJ are the VAS and ODI. Initial data from small cohorts offer promising results, although more data with more outcome measures are necessary.

References

1. Dworkin R, Turk D, Farrar J, et al. Core outcome measures for chronic pain clinical trials: IMMPACT recommendations. Pain. 2005;113(1–2):9–19. doi:10.1016/j.pain.2004.09.012
2. Hawker GA, Mian S, Kendzerska T, French M. Measures of adult pain: Visual Analog Scale for Pain (VAS Pain), Numeric Rating Scale for Pain (NRS Pain), McGill Pain Questionnaire (MPQ), Short-Form McGill Pain Questionnaire (SF-MPQ), Chronic Pain Grade Scale (CPGS), Short Form-36 Bodily Pain Scale (SF-36 BPS), and Measure of Intermittent and Constant Osteoarthritis Pain (ICOAP). Arthritis Care Res. 2011;63(Suppl 11):S240–S252. doi: 10.1002/acr.20543. PMID: 22588748.
3. Visual Analogue Scale. https://assessment-module.yale.edu/im-palliative/visual-analogue-scale
4. Kerns RD, Turk DC, Rudy TE. The West Haven-Yale Multidimensional Pain Inventory (WHYMPI). Pain. 1985;23(4):345–356. doi:10.1016/0304-3959(85)90004-1. PMID: 4088697.
5. Verra ML, Angst F, Staal JB, et al. Reliability of the Multidimensional Pain Inventory and stability of the MPI classification system in chronic back pain. BMC Musculoskelet Disord. 2012;13:155. doi:10.1186/1471-2474-13-155
6. Keller S, Bann CM, Dodd SL, et al. Validity of the Brief Pain Inventory for use in documenting the outcomes of patients with noncancer pain. Clin J Pain. 2004;20(5):309–318. doi:10.1097/00002508-200409000-00005. PMID: 15322437.
7. Cleeland CS, Ryan KM. Pain assessment: Global use of the Brief Pain Inventory. Ann Acad Med Singap. 1994;23(2):129–138. PMID: 8080219.
8. Pressure ulcer assessment and prevention in oncology settings: A review. https://www.researchgate.net/figure/Brief-pain-inventory-adapted-with-permission_fig1_216104815
9. Fairbank JC, Pynsent PB. The Oswestry Disability Index. Spine. 2000;25(22):2940–2952. doi:10.1097/00007632-200011150-00017. PMID: 11074683.
10. Sheng J, Liu S, Wang Y, et al. The link between depression and chronic pain: Neural mechanisms in the brain. Neural Plast. 2017;2017:9724371. doi:10.1155/2017
11. Beck AT, Ward CH, Mendelson M, et al. An inventory for measuring depression. Arch Gen Psychiatry. 1961;4(6):561–571. doi:10.1001/archpsyc.1961.01710120031004
12. Edwards JE, McQuay HJ, Moore RA, Collins SL. Reporting of adverse effects in clinical trials should be improved: Lessons from acute postoperative pain. J Pain Symptom Manag. 1999;18(6):427–437.
13. MiDAS ENCORE Study. https://clinicaltrials.gov/ct2/show/NCT02093520
14. Investigating Superion™ in Spinal Stenosis. https://clinicaltrials.gov/ct2/show/NCT00692276
15. Abou-Al-Shaar H, Adogwa O, Mehta AI. Lumbar spinal stenosis: Objective measurement scales and ambulatory status. Asian Spine J. 2018;12(4):765–774. doi:10.31616/asj.2018.12.4.765. PMID: 30060388; PMCID: PMC6068421.
16. Stucki G, Liang MH, Fossel AH, Katz JN. Relative responsiveness of condition-specific and generic health status measures in degenerative lumbar spinal stenosis. J Clin Epidemiol. 1995;48(11):1369–1378. doi:10.1016/0895-4356(95)00054-2. PMID: 7490600.
17. McConnell S, Kolopack P, Davis AM. The Western Ontario and McMaster Universities Osteoarthritis Index (WOMAC): A review of its utility and measurement properties. Arthritis Rheum. 2001;45:453–461. doi:10.1002/1529-0131(200110)45:5<453::AID-ART365>3.0.CO;2-W
18. Bellamy N. WOMAC Osteoarthritis Index: User guide IV. WOMAC, 2000.

19. Kim YH, Moon DE. Sacral nerve stimulation for the treatment of sacroiliac joint dysfunction: A case report. Neuromodulation. 2010;13(4):306–310. doi:10.1111/j.1525-1403.2009.00270.x. PMID: 21992888.
20. Goroszeniuk T. The effect of peripheral neuromodulation on pain from the sacroiliac joint: A retrospective cohort study. Neuromodulation. 2019;22(5):661–666. doi:10.1111/ner.12803. PMID: 30238573.
21. Chakrabortty S, Kumar S, Gupta D, Rudraraju S. Intractable sacroiliac joint pain treated with peripheral nerve field stimulation. J Anaesthesiol Clin Pharmacol. 2016;32(3):392–394. doi:10.4103/0970-9185.173336. PMID: 27625495; PMCID: PMC5009853.
22. Patil AA, Otto D, Raikar S. Peripheral nerve field stimulation for sacroiliac joint pain. Neuromodulation. 2014;17(1):98–101. doi:10.1111/ner.12030. PMID: 23441931.
23. Guentchev M, Preuss C, Rink R, et al. Long-term reduction of sacroiliac joint pain with peripheral nerve stimulation. Oper Neurosurg. 2017;13(5):634–639. doi:10.1093/ons/opx017. PMID: 28922873.
24. Comparison of Senza to Commercial Spinal Cord Stimulation for the Treatment of Chronic Pain. https://clinicaltrials.gov/ct2/show/NCT01609972
25. Guentchev M, Preuss C, Rink R, et al. Technical note: Treatment of sacroiliac joint pain with peripheral nerve stimulation. Neuromodulation. 2015;18(5):392–396. doi:10.1111/ner.12255. PMID: 25354279.

15

Complications of peripheral nerve stimulation for sacroiliac pain

Meghan Cantlon Hughes and Alaa Abd-Elsayed

Introduction

This chapter will look at complications of peripheral nerve stimulation (PNS) by stratifying them into three distinct categories: hardware-related complications, biologic complications, and programming or therapy-related complications.

History

In theory, PNS is very straightforward: It involves the application of electrical current (onto a peripheral nerve) for medical therapy. As is well documented, PNS emerged from the work of Drs. Campbell and Long at Johns Hopkins University in 1976.[1,2] Unfortunately, as with many things, what is simple in theory has been intensely complicated in practice.

PNS originated with large surface cuff electrodes, which were eventually refined when the ability to perform functional nerve mapping with the use of circumferential electrical stimulation was devised.[2] This technique provides for significantly improved targeting of sensory fascicles. Paddle electrodes were then eventually replaced by percutaneous cylindrical spinal cord stimulation (SCS) electrodes, which significantly expanded and improved the ability to target afferent sensory fibers as well as to reduce the complication rate.[3] The newest advances include radiofrequency needle probes, which allow doctors to induce paresthesia in patients who are awake in order to map the pain pattern and further guide treatment. Since the 1960s, not only have neuromodulation therapies improved people's lives, but they have improved themselves, becoming smaller, simpler to implant, and better able to target specific nerves and sites. They have also become more cost effective.

PNS did not truly "take off" until the late 1990s. The stagnation was secondary to nonstandardized surgical approaches that resulted in poor outcomes and multiple morbidities (rotation, torsion, and translation, among others). The result was often loss of the nerve fiber stimulation secondary to scarring. But in the late 1990s, PNS saw a surge of activity and expansion into the upper and lower extremities and the cranial, occipital, and lumbar nerves. These dynamic developments and changes were all driven by the introduction of percutaneous cylindrical SCS-type electrodes for use in PNS.[4] Essentially new techniques and new tools allowed electrical fields to be placed near the neural fascicles without the need for open dissection. These technological advancements represented a true marriage of engineering and medicine.

Today, PNS is one of the most rapidly growing segments of operative neuromodulation. It continues to evolve as current and emerging clinical indications become matched by basic and clinical research, technological developments, and procedural refinements. Neuromodulation is the fastest-growing segment of the overall medical device industry: The number of novel neuromodulation devices approved by the U.S. Food and Drug Administration grew 35% in 2007.[5]

Complications

Hardware-related complications

Hardware-related complications remain the most common PNS complications. These include lead migration or fracture, connection issues, and premature battery depletion.

As discussed, the complications of the early, nerve-dissection approach to PNS placement and therapy were numerous and significant and represented a primary factor in the overall lack of acceptance and use of PNS prior to 1999.

The first electrodes used by Wall and Sweet during their development of the "gate-control" theory were as basic as metal wires being inserted into the nerve or immediately adjacent to it.[6] Interestingly, at roughly the same time, Shelden et al. (~1960s) were using cuff electrodes for PNS,[7] which involved the use of a metal ring that wrapped around the nerve itself and provided stimulation. It should be no surprise that these techniques were associated with scarring around the nerve in question as well as the development of "fibrosis and nerve constriction from the lead itself."[6] These techniques also suffered from issues related to preferential nerve stimulation—only that part of the nerve directly in contact with the metal responded—which then led to issues related to larger nerves and paresthesia only occurring during contraction or relaxation or not occurring at all. The issue of preferential stimulation was overcome with the innovation of button-type electrodes.[8] The development of these small electrodes was welcome, but they had to be sutured to the perineurium of the portion of the nerve corresponding to the underlying sensory fascicles. This approach took time, expertise, and a great deal of nerve manipulation, all of which left it open to complications such as infection, scarring, and fibrosis.

Cuff electrodes faced the unique dilemma of nerve strangulation. In other words, despite the development of increasingly biocompatible materials,[7] nerve fibrosis or ischemia secondary to the electrode strangling the nerve within its soft tissue housing remained a primary concern. This complication was so insidious that it ultimately served as a primary impetus for the complete abandonment of these cuff devices.[9-11] In short, iatrogenic nerve injuries such as fibrosis and scarring were common prior to the development of the percutaneous approach, and the result was often complete loss of function due to nerve injury.[9,10]

Beyond fibrosis, scarring, and ultimate destruction of the nerve being treated loomed an even more problematic complication: lead migration, an issue that still haunts the PNS practitioner today. Meticulous dissection and secure suturing of cuff leads did not wholly alleviate the issue. Even more problematic is the fact that the only solution to lead migration is often complete revision of electrode placement, particularly in the older device design. Revision rates were reported to exceed 85%[11] prior to the inception of percutaneous lead placement.

Looking at the history of PNS, it becomes apparent that some of the technical complications have disappeared with technological advancements, while others remain essentially unchanged. What is clear is that since the advent of the percutaneous approach, most complications are now related to hardware: that is, lead migration and lead breakage.[12,13] Although lead migration remains common, it is also now much easier to fix, and a simple technique allows for repositioning without reopening the generator pocket.[14,15] Lead kinks or breaks typically occur at transition points over joints or traversing long distances or are due to excessive stretching or compression. The new devices designed specifically for PNS (vs. SCS devices being used off-label for PNS) are much more cognizant of lead length as well as tunneling length. These new devices are designed to sit almost anywhere on the body, and the need for extensive tunneling to a pocket location is now less common. Regardless, the practitioner should always be considering the path the lead will have to take to reach the pulse generator and take into account joint spaces or compression points it may traverse. All of this, of course, reduces the chances of both lead migration and lead breakage.

Biologic complications

The most common biologic complication is certainly infection of any kind. Although it is difficult to get a clear data point, infection rates seem to hover around 3%,[2] and infections can occur in both the short and long term. Poor surgical technique is likely the leading cause of surgical site infection. Utmost care should always be taken to create a sterile field and to maintain it throughout the surgery. The surgical site should be carefully cleaned prior to any interventions. Unfortunately, if an infection does occur, removal of the PNS device in its entirety is likely to be necessary. The patient will need to undergo systemic, appropriate antibiotic therapy to treat the infection. Often, the PNS device can be reimplanted several months after its initial removal.

Hemorrhages have been documented with PNS placement,[2] but they are rare and tend to be easy to control and treat since the device is placed in such a superficial location. If a hematoma does occur it is rarely symptomatic due to its location. "Wound dehiscence and erosion" are rare as well but have been documented.[16]

There have been documented issues related to pain over the site of hardware implantation. This is often transient or can be managed with relative ease.

Although extremely rare, biologic complications such as serious nerve damage and paralysis are possible.[17]

Programming and therapy-related complications

Programming and therapy-related complications are the least threatening of all possible complications and can typically be managed by addressing the device programming itself. They include either loss of the paresthesia or painful or unpleasant paresthesia. In rare situations, these issues may lead to device removal if the therapy is considered a failure.[17]

Other complications

Finally, there is an ongoing theoretical debate related to the possibility and concern of placing the PNS device into the wrong anatomic compartment. Data supports this being a theoretical versus legitimate concern. However, it is worth emphasizing that the placement of the electrode lead into the subcutaneous epifascial plane and its proximity to the nerve being stimulated is paramount. Without proper placement, paresthesia will not be achieved and the procedure will be moot. Today, most practitioners use fluoroscopy or intraoperative ultrasound to both localize the nerve and confirm lead placement.[13,18–20]

Conclusion

For many years, PNS was plagued by serious complications and procedural limitations. The original PNS procedural approach, which required nerve dissection and direct stimulation created a PNS history rife with permanent nerve fibrosis, scarring, and damage and revision rates exceeding 85%. It is no wonder PNS procedures failed to keep pace with more successful and safe therapies like SCS and intrathecal drug delivery.

The innovation of the percutaneous approach to PNS placement and procedure changed everything and created a landscape ripe for the launch of multiple new devices and techniques that transformed an obsolete procedural practice into an emerging, cutting-edge approach. Device innovation and development, paired with a growing need for preventive, minimally invasive procedures, has led PNS to quickly become a leading player in the field of chronic pain management.

Perhaps most importantly, the complications related to current PNS procedures are rare and minor. Hospital admission is exceedingly unlikely. Every new device on the market is working not only to improve performance but also to mitigate risks such as lead migration and infection. The horizon will be filled with devices with sleeker technology and design that are easier to implant and have a lower risk profile. Gone are the days when PNS procedures resulted in permanent nerve damage or a nearly guaranteed need for revision.

With the advent of these new devices has come the corresponding development of procedural approaches that minimize complications of any kinds and nearly eliminate serious complications. Together, these developments have changed the way we think about chronic pain management and prevention.

References

1. Campbell, J. N., & Long, D. M. Peripheral nerve stimulation in the treatment of intractable pain. *Journal of Neurosurgery* **45**, 692–699 (1976).

2. Slavin, K. V. History of peripheral nerve stimulation. *Progress in Neurological Surgery* **24**, 1–15 (2011).

3. Deer, T. R., Pope, J. E., & Kaplan, M. A novel method of neurostimulation of the peripheral nervous system: The StimRouter implantable device. *Techniques in Regional Anesthesia and Pain Management* **16**, 113–117 (2012).

4. Weiner, R. L., & Reed, K. L. Peripheral neurostimulation for control of intractable occipital neuralgia. *Neuromodulation* **2**, 217–221 (1999).

5. Lynch, C., & Lynch, Z. The Neurotechnology Industry 2007 Report: Drugs, devices and diagnostics for the brain and nervous system. *NeuroInsights* (2007).

6. Slavin, K. V. Technical Aspects of Peripheral Nerve Stimulation: Hardware and Complications. In Slavin (Ed.), *Peripheral nerve stimulation* Vol. 24 189–202 (Karger Publishers, 2011).

7. Shelden, C., Paul, F., Jacques, D., & Pudenz, R. Electrical stimulation of the nervous system. *Surgical Neurology* **4**, 127–132 (1975).

8. Nashold, B. S., Mullen, J. B., & Avery, R. Peripheral nerve stimulation for pain relief using a multicontact electrode system. *Journal of Neurosurgery* **51**, 872–873 (1979).

9. Nielson, K., Watts, C., & Clark, W. Peripheral nerve injury from implantation of chronic stimulating electrodes for pain control. *Surgical Neurology* **5**, 51–53 (1976).

10. Kirsch, W., Lewis, J., & Simon, R. Experiences with electrical stimulation devices for the control of chronic pain. *Medical Instrumentation* **9**, 217–220 (1975).

11. Nashold Jr, B., Goldner, J., Mullen, J., & Bright, D. Long-term pain control by direct peripheral-nerve stimulation. *Journal of Bone and Joint Surgery* **64**, 1–10 (1982).

12. Relief, C., Virginia, W., & Hayek, S. M. Occipital neurostimulation-induced muscle spasms: Implications for lead placement. *Pain Physician* **12**, 867–876 (2009).

13. Trentman, T. L., Dodick, D. W., Zimmerman, R. S., & Birch, B. D. Percutaneous occipital stimulator lead tip erosion: Report of 2 cases. *Pain Physician* **11**, 253–256 (2008).

14. Slavin, K. V., & Vannemreddy, P. S. Repositioning of supraorbital nerve stimulation electrode using retrograde needle insertion: A technical note. *Neuromodulation* **14**, 160–164 (2011).

15. Mammis, A., & Mogilner, A. Y. A technique of distal to proximal revision of peripheral neurostimulator leads. *Stereotactic and Functional Neurosurgery* **89**, 65–69 (2011).

16. Harland, T. A., Zbrzeski, C., DeMarzio, M., et al. Craniofacial peripheral nerve stimulation: Analysis of a single institution series. *Neuromodulation* **23**, 805–811 (2020).

17. Eldabe, S., Buchser, E., & Duarte, R. V. Complications of spinal cord stimulation and peripheral nerve stimulation techniques: A review of the literature. *Pain Medicine* **17**, 325–336 (2015).

18. Huntoon, M. A., & Burgher, A. H. Ultrasound-guided permanent implantation of peripheral nerve stimulation (PNS) system for neuropathic pain of the extremities: Original cases and outcomes. *Pain Medicine* **10**, 1369–1377 (2009).

19. Carayannopoulos, A., Beasley, R., & Sites, B. Facilitation of percutaneous trial lead placement with ultrasound guidance for peripheral nerve stimulation trial of ilioinguinal neuralgia: A technical note. *Neuromodulation* **12**, 296–301 (2009).

20. Skaribas, I., & Aló, K. Ultrasound imaging and occipital nerve stimulation. *Neuromodulation* **13**, 126–130 (2010).

PART V

Surgical fusion for the sacroiliac joint

16

Patient selection

Sarafina Kankam, Gregory Lawson Smith, and
Johnathan Goree

Introduction

Fusion of the sacroiliac joint (SIJ) was first described by Smith-Petersen and Rogers in
the *Journal of Bone and Joint Surgery* in 1921, when they described an open posterolateral
transiliac approach.[1] Open surgical approaches can provide pain relief, but recovery times
are long and the complication rate is high.[2] Therefore, open fusion of the SIJ is commonly
reserved for pelvic ring fractures in the setting of trauma, adjunctive treatment for SIJ infection, or management of sacral tumors, or when performed as part of a multi-segmental
long fusion for spinal deformities.[3,4]

Over the past century, this technique has evolved into multiple minimally invasive
lateral techniques. In 2008 the U.S. Food and Drug Administration (FDA) approved the
first minimally invasive device for SIJ fusion, which marked the beginning of increased use
of the minimally invasive surgical technique.[3] Recent clinical trial evidence suggests that
minimally invasive SIJ fusion can provide superior pain relief, functional outcomes, and
better quality of life compared to nonsurgical management in select patients.[5] Graham-
Smith et al. conducted the first multicenter comparative cohort study to determine differences in outcomes between open and minimally invasive surgical techniques and found a
significant difference in operating time, estimated blood loss, and hospital length of stay.[6]
Hospital stays were reduced by nearly 4 days, and operating time was on average 1.5 hours
shorter in the minimally invasive surgery cohort. Improvement in pain was also clinically
and statistically significant, with minimally invasive surgery patients scoring on average 3
points lower on the visual analog scale (VAS) compared to those who underwent traditional
open SIJ fusion (−6.2 vs. −2.7 points).[6]

By 2012, over 80% of SIJ fusions were performed with a minimally invasive technique. Over the past 3 to 5 years, with multiple new percutaneous techniques, the number
of SIJ fusions is continually increasing.[6] While percutaneous and minimally invasive techniques have decreased risks compared to other SIJ fusion modalities, these procedures still
carry higher risks than injections or radiofrequency ablations. In a review published by

Shamrock et al., 11% of minimally invasive SIJ fusion cases resulted in a procedure-related complication. The most common was surgical wound infection/drainage, but other complications included nerve root impingement, trochanteric bursitis, hematoma formation, and hairline fracture of the ilium.[2]

Due to the risks of this intervention and the challenges in diagnosis of SIJ pain, patient selection is paramount. In this chapter, we will provide a literature review of the evidence behind proper patient selection for minimally invasive fusion of the SIJ.

Indications for surgery

Both the International Society for the Advancement of Spine Surgery (ISASS) and the North American Spine Society (NASS) have issued patient selection recommendations and insurance coverage criteria for SIJ fusion surgery.[7,8] For SIJ fusion to be considered medically necessary and for positive predictive surgical outcomes, the following should be evident:

- Patients should be diagnosed with SIJ pain. Thus, confirmation that the SIJ is the main pain generator is of utmost importance to help ensure that patients receive benefit from the procedure. Additional or alternative diagnoses that could be responsible for the patient's ongoing pain or disability should be investigated and ruled out.[9]
- SIJ dysfunction that is the direct result of SIJ disruption or degenerative sacroiliitis (can include patients whose symptoms began in pregnancy or postpartum and have persisted for >6 months). This also includes acute, non-acute, and non-traumatic fractures involving the SIJ.[10]
- Persistent moderate to severe pain and functional impairment, usually at least 5 out of 10 on the pain scale[11]
- Specific physical examination findings, including tenderness to palpation over the posterior aspect of the joint and the sacral sulcus (Fortin's point)[8]
- Positive findings on at least three out of five SIJ provocation physical examination maneuvers[12,13]
- Must fail to respond to at least 6 months of conservative, nonoperative management such as medical management, physical therapy, fluoroscopy-guided injections, and/or radiofrequency ablations
- Should have at least 50% reduction in pain after a fluoroscopically guided injection of local anesthetic into the SIJ[11]

Contraindications

Minimally invasive SIJ fusion is contraindicated in certain circumstances. This procedure should be avoided in patients with deformities or anatomic variations that prevent or interfere with device placement, tumor of sacral or iliac bone, active infection at the treatment site, unstable fracture of the sacrum or ilium involving the SIJ, and allergy or intolerance to metal or any of the implant components.[14]

Minimally invasive SIJ fusion is also not indicated for patients who have had less than 6 months of SIJ pain, failure to pursue conservative measures (unless contraindicated), pain that is not confirmed with response to intraarticular SIJ injections, or the presence of other pathology that would prevent the patient from deriving benefit from SIJ fusion.[7]

Imaging

There are several imaging modalities a provider can use to ascertain the integrity of the SIJ when fusion is being considered. These include plain radiography, magnetic resonance imaging (MRI), computed tomography (CT), and bone scintigraphy. However, these imaging studies serve more to exclude other causes of pain rather than to diagnose idiopathic SIJ pain.[13] The NASS states that diagnostic imaging studies should include the following:[8]

- Imaging (plain radiographs and a CT or MRI) of the SIJ that excludes the presence of destructive lesions (tumor, infection) or inflammatory arthropathy that would not be properly addressed by percutaneous SIJ fusion
- Imaging of the pelvis (anteroposterior [AP] plain radiograph) to rule out concomitant hip pathology
- Imaging of the lumbar spine (CT or MRI) to rule out neural compression or other degenerative condition that can be causing low back or buttock pain

Surgical approaches to minimally invasive SIJ fusion

There are multiple surgical approaches for minimally invasive SIJ fusion. The two most common are the lateral and posterior approaches. According to the literature, both the lateral and posterior placements of the implants have similar performance in terms of SIJ stability.[16] Subsequent chapters of this book detail the surgical techniques, safety, and efficacy of the two approaches.

Minimally invasive lateral fusion

The majority of the literature regarding minimally invasive SIJ fusion is based on this approach, although the evidence for the posterior approach is increasing. The lateral approach to SIJ fusion was approved by the FDA in 2008.[3] This approach to SIJ fusion is generally performed by surgeons. The surgery involves dissecting through the lateral gluteus musculature down to the ileum and then inserting a device to transfix the ilium and sacrum together across the SIJ. This approach carries a higher risk of neurologic damage to the lumbosacral nerve roots.[11]

Minimally invasive posterior fusion

The posterior approach is a newer technique that has paved a pathway for interventional pain physicians to offer this therapy in lieu of strictly surgeons.[11] The posterior approach is performed through a dorsal midline or paramedian incision with dissection to the dorsal ligamentous recess between the sacrum and ilium; the soft tissues of the joint are then debrided, and an implant and bone graft material are placed.[17] An advantage of the posterior approach compared to the lateral approach is that it is less invasive and fewer muscles are disrupted during the procedure. Posterior access also provides better visibility, especially when treating larger patients.[18]

Other patient considerations

Psychiatric history

It is recommended that patients who are being considered for SIJ fusion should not be diagnosed with generalized pain behavior or generalized pain disorders such as somatoform disorder or fibromyalgia.[19] Many providers use the same standards they would for other spinal fusion surgeries or for implanting neuromodulation systems used to treat pain. Studies have shown that presurgical somatization, in particular, was associated with poor response (i.e., less treatment-related benefit) to lumbar surgery and spinal cord stimulation.[20] Pain is associated with depression and anxiety, and symptoms of preoperative anxiety and depression occur in approximately one-third of patients with chronic back pain undergoing surgery.[21] In most patients, once their pain has improved after surgery, their depression also improves. Several risk factors have been identified that correlate with greater risk for unsuccessful outcomes from pain treatment, including pain chronicity, psychological distress, pain-related catastrophizing, a history of abuse or trauma, nicotine use and substance abuse history, poor social support, and significant cognitive deficits.[22] It is important to assess each patient's psychiatric history and current psychiatric symptoms, weigh the benefits and the risks of the procedure, and then use clinical judgment before proceeding with surgery.

Bone density

The relationship between sacral bone density and surgical outcomes of SIJ fusion is an important consideration. It is particularly crucial to understand the relationship between bone quality or density and the effectiveness of the surgical technique from a biomechanical perspective.[16] Bone mineral density (BMD) is a good preoperative indicator of sacral screw-fixation strength.[23] Sacral-sided loosening of a sacroiliac fusion appears to be the most common mode of failure. The implant loosening or failure often occurs due to poor bone quality in the sacrum area.[24] Osteoporosis is a relative contraindication, since this condition may limit the degree of obtainable correction, stabilization, and/or the amount of mechanical fixation.[25] A dual energy x-ray absorptiometry (DEXA) scan measures BMD and is used to diagnose osteoporosis, defined as a bone density below a score of −2.5. Development of an accessible method for evaluating sacral bone density would be instrumental in determining the relation of bone density to successful SIJ and lumbosacral fixation and fusion.[24]

As mentioned previously in this chapter, CT is an imaging modality that is sometimes used to rule out other etiologies of pain in patients being evaluated for SIJ dysfunction prior to surgery. Currently, research has shown that direct Hounsfield unit (HU) measurements from diagnostic CT scans have the potential to be used opportunistically for osteoporosis screening.[26] As it relates to SIJ fusion, opportunistic CT scans can be employed to evaluate sacral CT attenuation and predict sacral BMD, which can aid in patient selection.[24] At this time, more research is needed to identify what these HU thresholds would be at specific anatomic regions.[26]

Previous lumbar spinal fusion

Patients with previous lumbar spinal fusion may present with SIJ dysfunction. The prevalence range of SIJ pain in patients who have undergone lumbosacral fusion is 43% to 61%.[27]

In this patient population, it can be difficult to discern the etiology of their pain. The presence of concomitant symptomatic lumbar dysfunction can potentially confound the treatment effect. Once SIJ pain has been established as the primary pain generator in these patients, they can also undergo SIJ fusion. A study by Rudolf highlighted that patients with a history of prior lumbar spinal fusion reported a slightly greater satisfaction with SIJ fusion when compared to patients with no history of spinal fusion or patients being treated nonsurgically for lumbar pathology.[28] Regardless of whether they had undergone prior lumbar spinal fusion or no previous spinal fusion, the patients in the study still demonstrated a statistically and clinically significant improvement in pain after minimally invasive SIJ fusion.[28]

Smoking history

It is important to optimize the condition of patients preceding surgery. Tobacco cessation for at least 4 to 6 weeks prior to surgery is recommended. A pooled patient-level analysis of two multicenter randomized controlled trials and one multicenter single-arm prospective trial by Dengler et al. found that current smokers who underwent SIJ fusion had reduced pain response (by 5.9 VAS points) and higher disability levels than nonsmokers who had undergone SIJ fusion.[29] Smoking cessation also reduces comorbidities and can decrease complication rates after spine surgery.[30]

Diabetes history

It is also recommended that patients with a history of diabetes have their hemoglobin A1C (HbA1c) controlled prior to surgery. There are no evidence-based guidelines published that preclude surgery in patients above a particular HbA1c value; however, most guidelines advise that a safe target for elective orthopedic surgery is below 8 to 9.[31] Glucose management is important as hyperglycemia can result in surgical site infection, poor wound healing, increased risk of pulmonary embolism, and other comorbidities.[32]

Long-term effects

For carefully selected patients, SIJ fusion is overall a safe, successful, and well-tolerated procedure. If patients have benefit from SIJ fusion surgery, the surgery appears durable through 5 years.[33] Surgical revision is a key outcome for implants. Cher et al. looked at the 4-year revision rate for SIJ fusions in a study that included 11,388 patients from 2009 to 2014. The cumulative 4-year revision rate was 3.5%, meaning that 96.5% of the fusions were free from revision, also known as survivorship. The survivorship rate for SIJ implants is high and improving, as the revision rate has decreased annually since 2009. The revision rate for SIJ fusions is about the same or somewhat higher than that of total hip replacements (<2–4% 4-year revision rate) but lower than that of lumbar spine procedures (the 4-year revision rate for lumbar decompression is 10.6–17.2% and the 4-year revision rate for lumbar fusion is 10.7–13.5%).[34]

Conclusion

While SIJ fusion has shown efficacy for pain generated from the SIJ, patient selection is of utmost importance. First, a thorough physical examination must be conducted to ensure that the SIJ is indeed the pain generator of interest. Second, imaging is indicated to rule out other common pathology, including spinal stenosis, lumbar radiculopathy, post-laminectomy syndrome, and hip arthropathy. Lastly, patient optimization is key. Comorbidities like diabetes, depression, history of smoking, and osteoporosis should be identified and included in the risk/benefit analysis prior to the procedure. If delaying the procedure is possible in order to decrease risks and improve chances for success, this should be considered.

References

1. Smith-Petersen MN. Arthrodesis of the sacroiliac joint: A new method of approach. *J Bone Joint Surg.* 1921;3:400–405.
2. Shamrock AG, Patel A, Alam M, et al. The safety profile of percutaneous minimally invasive sacroiliac joint fusion. *Global Spine J.* 2019;9(8):874–880. doi:10.1177/2192568218816981
3. Lorio MP, Polly DW Jr, Ninkovic I, et al. Utilization of minimally invasive surgical approach for sacroiliac joint fusion in surgeon population of ISASS and SMISS membership. *Open Orthop J.* 2014;8:1–6. doi:10.2174/1874325001408010001
4. BlueCross BlueShield of North Carolina. Corporate medical policy: Sacroiliac joint fusion/stabilization, May 2020. https://www.bluecrossnc.com/sites/default/files/document/attachment/services/public/pdfs/medicalpolicy/sacroiliac_joint_fusion_stabilization.pdf
5. Polly DW, Cher DJ, Wine KD, et al. Randomized controlled trial of minimally invasive sacroiliac joint fusion using triangular titanium implants vs nonsurgical management for sacroiliac joint dysfunction: 12-month outcomes. *Neurosurgery.* 2015;77(5):674–691. doi:10.1227/NEU.0000000000000988
6. Smith AG, Capobianco R, Cher D, et al. Open versus minimally invasive sacroiliac joint fusion: A multicenter comparison of perioperative measures and clinical outcomes. *Ann Surg Innov Res.* 2013;7(1):14. doi:10.1186/1750-1164-7-14
7. International Society for Advancement of Spine Surgery (ISASS). ISASS policy 2016 update: Minimally invasive sacroiliac joint fusion. https://www.isass.org/public-policy/isass-policy-statement-minimally-invasive-sacroiliac-joint-fusion-july-2016/
8. North American Spine Society (NASS). NASS coverage policy recommendations: Percutaneous sacroiliac joint fusion, June 9, 2015.
9. Lorio MP, Rashbaum R. ISASS policy statement—minimally invasive sacroiliac joint fusion. *Int J Spine Surg.* 2014;8:25. doi:10.14444/1025

10. iFuse treatments: Patient safety information. https://si-bone.com/si-joint-pain-treatment/ifuse-implant-system/risks

11. Falowski S, Sayed D, Pope J, et al. A review and algorithm in the diagnosis and treatment of sacroiliac joint pain. *J Pain Res.* 2020;13:3337–3348. doi:10.2147/JPR.S279390

12. Kokmeyer DJ, Van der Wurff P, Aufdemkampe G, Fickenscher TC. The reliability of multitest regimens with sacroiliac pain provocation tests. *J Manip Physiol Ther.* 2002;25(1):42–48. doi:10.1067/mmt.2002.120418

13. Laslett M, Aprill CN, McDonald B, Young SB. Diagnosis of sacroiliac joint pain: Validity of individual provocation tests and composites of tests. *Man Ther.* 2005;10(3):207–218. doi:10.1016/j.math.2005.01.003

14. iFuse patient surgery guide. https://si-bone.com/support/patient-resource-library/patient-surgery-guide

15. Dreyfuss P, Dreyer SJ, Cole A, Mayo K. Sacroiliac joint pain. *J Am Acad Orthop Surg.* 2004;12(4):255–265. doi:10.5435/00124635-200407000-00006

16. Joukar A, Kiapour A, Elgafy H, et al. Biomechanics of the sacroiliac joint: Surgical treatments. *Int J Spine Surg.* 2020;14(3):355–367. doi:10.14444/7047

17. Martin CT, Haase L, Lender PA, Polly DW. Minimally invasive sacroiliac joint fusion: The current evidence. *Int J Spine Surg.* 2020;14(Suppl 1):20–29. doi:10.14444/6072

18. Medtronic. Treatment options: SI joint fusion. https://www.medtronic.com/us-en/patients/treatments-therapies/sacroiliac-joint-fusion/treatment-options/si-fusion.html#

19. iFuse. Learn: What criteria must be met to qualify for SI joint fusion surgery? https://si-bone.com/si-joint-faqs/what-criteria-must-be-met-to-qualify-for-si-joint-fusion-surgery

20. Celestin J, Edwards RR, Jamison RN. Pretreatment psychosocial variables as predictors of outcomes following lumbar surgery and spinal cord stimulation: A systematic review and literature synthesis. *Pain Med.* 2009;10(4):639–653. doi:10.1111/j.1526-4637.2009.00632.x

21. Strøm J, Bjerrum MB, Nielsen CV, et al. Anxiety and depression in spine surgery: A systematic integrative review. *Spine J.* 2018;18(7):1272–1285. doi:10.1016/j.spinee.2018.03.017

22. Campbell CM, Jamison RN, Edwards RR. Psychological screening/phenotyping as predictors for spinal cord stimulation. *Curr Pain Headache Rep.* 2013;17(1):307. doi:10.1007/s11916-012-0307-6

23. Lu WW, Zhu Q, Holmes AD, et al. Loosening of sacral screw fixation under in vitro fatigue loading. *J Orthop Res.* 2000;18(5):808–814. doi:10.1002/jor.1100180519

24. Hoel RJ, Ledonio CG, Takahashi T, Polly DW Jr. Sacral bone mineral density (BMD) assessment using opportunistic CT scans. *J Orthop Res.* 2017;35(1):160–166. doi:10.1002/jor.23362

25. Zimmer Biomet. TriCor™ sacroiliac joint fusion system surgical technique guide. https://www.zimmerbiomet.com/content/dam/zimmer-biomet/medical-professionals/000-surgical-techniques/spine/tri-cor-sacroiliac-joint-fusion-system-surgical-technique-guide.pdf

26. Gausden EB, Nwachukwu BU, Schreiber JJ, et al. Opportunistic use of CT imaging for osteoporosis screening and bone density assessment: A qualitative systematic review. *J Bone Joint Surg Am.* 2017;99(18):1580–1590. doi:10.2106/JBJS.16.00749

27. DePalma MJ, Ketchum JM, Saullo TR. Etiology of chronic low back pain in patients having undergone lumbar fusion. *Pain Med.* 2011;12(5):732–739. doi:10.1111/j.1526-4637.2011.01098.x

28. Rudolf L. MIS fusion of the SI joint: Does prior lumbar spinal fusion affect patient outcomes? *Open Orthop J.* 2013;7:163–168. doi:10.2174/1874325001307010163

29. Dengler J, Duhon B, Whang P, et al. Predictors of outcome in conservative and minimally invasive surgical management of pain originating from the sacroiliac joint: A pooled analysis. *Spine.* 2017;42(21):1664–1673. doi:10.1097/BRS.0000000000002169

30. Berman D, Oren JH, Bendo J, Spivak J. The effect of smoking on spinal fusion. *Int J Spine Surg.* 2017;11(4):29. doi:10.14444/4029

31. Dhatariya K, Levy N, Kilvert A, et al. NHS diabetes guideline for the perioperative management of the adult patient with diabetes. *Diabet Med.* 2012;29(4):420–433. doi:10.1111/j.1464-5491.2012.03582.x

32. Akiboye F, Rayman G. Management of hyperglycemia and diabetes in orthopedic surgery. *Curr Diab Rep*. 2017;17(2):13. doi:10.1007/s11892-017-0839-6

33. Whang PG, Darr E, Meyer SC, et al. Long-term prospective clinical and radiographic outcomes after minimally invasive lateral transiliac sacroiliac joint fusion using triangular titanium implants. *Med Devices)*. 2019;12:411–422. doi:10.2147/MDER.S219862

34. Cher DJ, Reckling WC, Capobianco RA. Implant survivorship analysis after minimally invasive sacroiliac joint fusion using the iFuse Implant System(*). *Med Devices*. 2015;8:485–492. doi:10.2147/MDER.S94885

17

Surgical instrumentation

Nomen Azeem

Introduction

As with any surgical procedure, access to the appropriate surgical instrumentation is imperative for a safe and successful outcome. The development of minimally invasive surgeries helped to mitigate risk factors and complications at times associated with traditional open surgical procedure. The original sacroiliac joint (SIJ) fusion procedure was introduced in 1921 and was an open procedure.[1] Since 2008 the field has seen the development, market release, and adoption of two minimally invasive approaches developed for SIJ fusion, a posterior approach and a lateral approach. There are currently more than 20 SIJ fusion systems on the market. Minimally invasive SIJ fusion is not an open procedure in which the clinician may directly visualize anatomy; rather, it is a procedure guided by fluoroscopy or computed tomography (CT). Fluoroscopy is a type of medical imaging that shows a continuous x-ray image on a monitor. During a fluoroscopy-guided procedure, an x-ray beam is passed through the body and transmitted to a monitor to visualize bone and joint anatomy. In a CT scan, a series of x-ray images taken from different angles are combined to produce a more detailed image than a fluoroscopic image.

Patient positioning and preparation

The patient must be positioned appropriately on a radiolucent table for the duration of the procedure. The proper position for SIJ fusion must minimize lordosis of the lumbar spine, which can be accomplished with a Wilson frame. Kyphosis induced with a Wilson frame significantly increased flexion at L4–5 and L5–S1 by 47% and 21%, respectively, and it was found that the surgical technique of inducing kyphosis with the Wilson frame prior to incision significantly optimized exposure.[2] If a Wilson frame is not accessible, then a bump (i.e., gel bump or rolled-up towels) underneath the abdomen may be used.

Once the patient is positioned properly, the skin overlying the intended surgical site must be sterilized. The first use of an antiseptic skin agent in surgery is credited to the English surgeon Joseph Lister (1827–1912). Prior to the mid-19th century, limb amputation was associated with an alarming 50% postoperative mortality from sepsis. Lister began treating wounds with carbolic acid (phenol) in an effort to prevent tissue decay and the resultant infectious complications. As a result, the incidence of surgical sepsis fell dramatically, catalyzing the adoption of modern antiseptic techniques, including instrument sterilization, the use of surgical scrub and rubber gloves, and sterile patient preparation.[3,4] The antiseptic skin preparations most commonly used today are iodophors and chlorhexidine gluconate. In the case of the SIJ fusion, the lumbosacral area on the side designated for SIJ fusion must be prepped. A proper sterile field must be established using sterile towels and sterile drapes, and Incise drape (i.e., Ioban) may be used to protect against skin flora contamination.

Nonsurgical items for SIJ fusion procedure

During any surgical procedure, tools in addition to surgical instrumentation are necessary for planning, administration of local anesthetic, absorption of blood or fluid, infection prevention, and wound dressing. To begin, a sterile marking pen may be used to mark the skin for planned guide pin entry point and/or incision. A radiopaque pointer can be used under fluoroscopy to identify the intended needle, guide pin, and/or scalpel entry point. To anesthetize the skin prior to needle entry or incision, a skin needle (i.e., 25 gauge, 1.5 inches) with a syringe (10 cc) should be available. Local anesthetic (with or without epinephrine) is used to anesthetize the skin and underlying tissue for needle entry and incision; epinephrine has been shown to assist with hemostasis.[5] A spinal needle (i.e., 22 gauges, 3.5 inches) is often used to provide local anesthetic along the intended trajectory of the guide pin (Figure 17.1). Ray-tecs or sterile sponges are often used to absorb fluids and may be used to hold pressure for hemostasis. Normal saline (with or without antibiotic) should be available and can be used to irrigate the surgical wound prior to wound closure. Lastly, sterile dressing (i.e., Steri-Strips, gauze, Tegaderm) should be available to provide the surgical incision with a physical barrier from environmental elements and may absorb any residual postsurgical fluid.

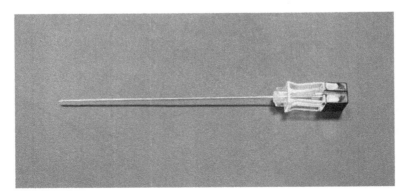

FIGURE 17.1. Spinal needle.

Surgical instruments for SIJ fusion procedure

The pertinent surgical instruments that should be supplied by the facility for SIJ fusion should allow for incising/dissecting, hemostasis, handling of instruments provided by the vendor, and surgical wound closure (Table 17.1). Although this chapter discusses the most common surgical instruments needed to complete the SIJ fusion, surgeon preference will also dictate which types of surgical instruments are used.

Cutting and dissecting

To begin the surgical procedure, instruments for cutting and dissecting must be available. Scalpels are used to cut superficial tissue and for cutdown to prepare a path for the dilator cannula in the trajectory of the guide pin[6] (Figure 17.2). The use of electrosurgery for cutting and dissecting is a surgeon's preference. High-frequency electrosurgery is commonly used in the operating room for cutting and dissecting of tissue. There are two types of electrocautery devices, bipolar and monopolar. In bipolar electrocautery current flows from one side of the forceps through the tissue and then back through the other side of the forceps and to the generator. In monopolar electrocautery, a pen-type instrument is used to deliver current to the tissue, which is then returned to the generator through an adhesive grounding pad placed on the skin proximal to the surgical work area.

TABLE 17.1 Surgical instruments required for SIJ fusion, provided by facility

Surgical instrument	Use	Types
Scalpel	Incision of superficial tissue	▪ #10 blade: larger skin incision ▪ #11 blade: stab incision ▪ #15 blade: finer skin incision
Electrosurgery	Dissection of deeper tissue/coagulation	▪ Bipolar ▪ Monopolar
Sponge clamps	Hold guide pin	
Forceps	Hold skin edges, needles	▪ Adson: with or without teeth; most commonly used ▪ Debakey: longer, more delicate; no teeth
Needle holder	Hold suture needle	▪ Large ▪ Small
Orthopedic mallet	Advance guide pin, dilators, broach, implant	▪ Not a "hammer" ▪ Can also be used as a pusher or reduction device
Orthopedic drill	Clear path for implant, stimulate bone growth	▪ Battery operated ▪ Drill bit provided in kit
Suture	Incision closure	▪ Absorbable ▪ Nonabsorbable
Suture scissors	Cut suture	▪ Mayo ▪ Straight = "suture scissors" used to cut suture

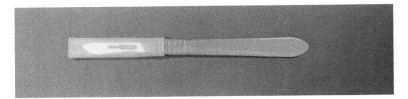

FIGURE 17.2. Scalpel.

Management of bleeding

All procedures requiring an incision will require instruments to appropriately manage bleeding from the incision or surgical wound. Suction is often used to remove excess fluid, blood, and debris within and/or around the incision. Suction may also be used during dissection for better visualization and during wound closure as necessary. Electrosurgery if available can be used for coagulation with forceps (bipolar) or pen-type instrument (monopolar). If hemostasis is a challenge, thrombin Gelfoam sponges may be used for coagulation. Thrombin Gelfoam is a sterile sponge consisting of water-insoluble porous pliable purified pork skin gelatin USP granules that can be cut and placed in a bleeding wound.

SIJ fusion placement

After the incision has been made and bleeding has been managed, the placement of the SIJ fusion begins. At this point during surgery, along with the prepacked kit provided by the device manufacturer, there must be additional surgical instruments provided by the facility. Sponge clamps (ring forceps) may be used to hold the guide pin outside of the x-ray field in order to limit surgeon's concentrated radiation exposure[6] (Figure 17.3). An orthopedic mallet is necessary for this procedure in order to advance the guide pin, dilators, broach, and implant delivery device[6] (Figure 17.4). An orthopedic drill may be necessary for certain posterior fusion approaches to clear out the intended path for the implant and to stimulate

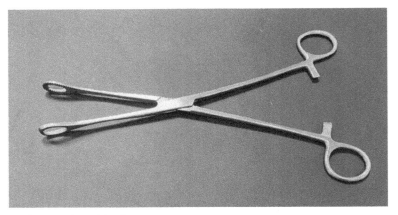

FIGURE 17.3. Sponge clamp/ring forceps.

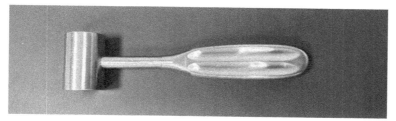

FIGURE 17.4. Orthopedic mallet.

bone growth for a robust fusion. In certain lateral approaches, an orthopedic drill may be used to drill the guide pin from the lateral ilium through the SIJ or to place screws.

Wound closure

Effective wound closure is imperative for a successful surgical outcome and to prevent infection. To close a surgical wound, forceps ("pickups") are necessary to hold the skin edges of the incision and to grasp the suture needle during the suturing process (Figure 17.5). A needle holder is used to hold the suture needle during the suturing process and for instrument tie (Figure 17.6). Typically for an SIJ fusion incision, a two-layer closure is recommended. An absorbable braided suture such as Vicryl is used to approximate deep tissue, followed by either an absorbable monofilament suture such as Monocryl or surgical staples for skin closure (Figure 17.7). Suture scissors are necessary to cut the sutures (Figure 17.8).

Instruments provided by the manufacturer

The SIJ fusion kits will vary per device manufacturer and approach (posterior or lateral) and will include the tools necessary to complete the SIJ fusion procedure. The surgical instruments provided in the prepacked kits have many similarities. The majority of the SIJ fusion systems on the market use a guide pin to enter the SIJ; dilators or cannulas can be placed over it in order to enter and expand the SIJ. Decorticators (broaches) are provided to clear a path for the intended implant as well as to stimulate bone growth. Certain manufacturers provide a drill bit to be used with an orthopedic drill to stimulate bone growth. Most of the SIJ fusion manufacturers provide a type of slap hammer to remove the dilators that are wedged into a tight space. Lastly, a fusion delivery system is provided to place the SIJ fusion device.

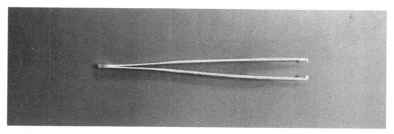

FIGURE 17.5. Forceps ("pickups").

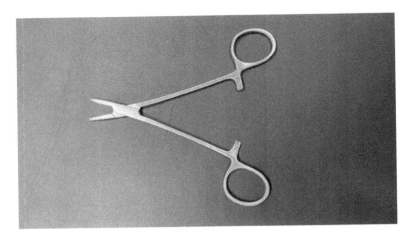

FIGURE 17.6. Needle holder.

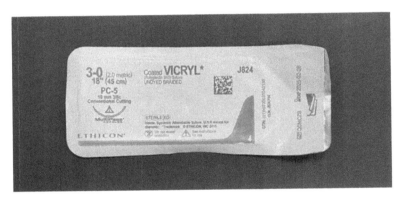

FIGURE 17.7. Suture.

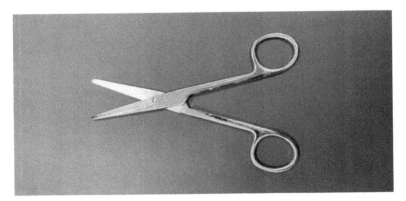

FIGURE 17.8. Suture scissors.

References

1. Smith-Peterson MN. Arthrodesis of the sacroiliac joint. A new method approach. J Bone Joint Surg Am. 1921;3:400–405.
2. Cardoso M, Rosner M. Does the Wilson frame assist with optimizing surgical exposure for minimally invasive lumbar fusions? J Neurosurg. 2010;28(5):E20–#21.
3. Hmani M, Lepor H. Skin preparation for the prevention of surgical site infection: Which agent is best? Rev Urol. 2009;11(4):190–195.
4. Newsom BD. Surgical wound infections: A historical review. Int J Infect Control. 2008;4:1.
5. Dunlevy T, O'Malley T, Postma G. Optimal concentration of epinephrine for vasoconstriction in neck surgery. Laryngoscope. 1996;106(11):1412–1414.
6. Kotb S. Surgical instruments. 2015. https://www.researchgate.net/publication/273001861

18

Preoperative considerations

Kenneth Fiala, Joshua Martens, and Alaa Abd-Elsayed

Introduction

In order to ensure the best outcome for any surgical procedure, it is essential to have a successful preoperative plan. In approximately 13% to 30% of patients with lower back pain, the pain is due to the sacroiliac joint (SIJ).[1-4] The preoperative considerations for SIJ fusion are centered around a thorough review of patient history and underlying risk factors, a well-reviewed procedural plan, and effective management of the patient's risk of infection and bleeding risk via anticoagulation.

A thorough review of the patient's history, combined with a complete physical exam, is essential to both confirm that the patient's pain arises from the SIJ and to identify any underlying conditions that may complicate the procedure or require further consultation with additional physicians. Prior to consideration for surgery, patients typically have completed nonsurgical management efforts including physical therapy per American Physical Therapy Association guidelines, intraarticular SIJ steroid injections, oral analgesics, and radiofrequency ablation of sacral nerve roots, without improvement in pain and dysfunction.[2,5] SIJ fusion will not improve a patient's condition if the pain is secondary to inflammatory conditions or is referred from other lumbar etiologies.[6,7] A physical exam should include full musculoskeletal and neurologic exam of the lumbar spine and bilateral lower extremities as well as a series of range-of-motion assessments of the joint.[8] A review of patient history should include comorbidities such as diabetes, cardiac disease, renal dysfunction, chronic edema, and methicillin-resistant Staphylococcus aureas (MRSA).[9] A complete medication review should also be completed, with specific focus on patient adherence to any active anticoagulation medications. Other health conditions and risk factors can be reviewed that may impact a patient's ability to assume the position necessary for the procedure or may prevent appropriate visualization of the surgical area, such as scar tissue from prior procedures. Additional consultations should take place preoperatively when necessary, and a repeat evaluation must be completed just prior to the procedure to confirm that the patient has adhered to preoperative instructions and to assess for any changes in medications and conditions.

Candidate selection

A good candidate for SIJ fusion is one who has completed all appropriate nonsurgical management efforts, including physical therapy, intraarticular SIJ steroid injections, oral analgesics, and radiofrequency ablation of sacral nerve roots, without improvement in pain.[2,5] Candidates should have a structured physical exam completed that includes documentation of the Fortin finger test, tenderness to palpation of the posterior superior iliac spine, posterior thigh thrust, flexion abduction external rotation test, pelvic gapping, pelvic compression, Gaenslen's test, and sacral thrust.[10] Candidates for surgery should also undergo a guided diagnostic block of the SIJ resulting in greater than 50% relief of symptoms.[10]

To further rule out confounding pain sources, additional actions should be taken. While patient history and physical exam may be sufficient to rule out concomitant hip pain, diagnostic hip injection should be used in cases of ambiguity.[10] Axial imaging and, if abnormal, epidural steroid injections, selective nerve root blocks, or facet injections may be used to rule out concomitant spine pain; however, this process is less reliable than the established process for hip pain.[10] Although not mandatory, patients can undergo a psychological evaluation prior to surgery, as poorly controlled psychological disorders may present an additional confounding factor and limit the potential benefit of intervention. Patients with underlying surgical risk factors such as chronic use of anticoagulants should proceed with caution, with appropriate management of anticoagulants preoperatively and postoperatively to minimize both surgical risk and the risk of abstaining from anticoagulant medications.

Ultimately, patients should undergo surgery if the treating physicians determine that the potential benefit of intervention outweighs the potential risks.

Surgical approaches

Two general techniques can be used to obtain arthrodesis of the SIJ: an open approach and a minimally invasive surgical (MIS) approach. The open approach can also be completed using an anterior approach. The MIS approach can be completed either posteriorly or can be transiliac (lateral approach). Patients who underwent SIJ fusion surgery via the MIS approach had better pain relief and perioperative surgical measures than those who underwent the open approach.[11,12]

Anticoagulation

While it is unlikely to encounter major vessels during the SIJ fusion procedure, regardless of approach, it is important to maintain a comprehensive knowledge of the local anatomy in order to minimize the risk of excessive bleeding. It is also important to appropriately manage patients who are actively taking anticoagulants, confirming that the patients have followed preoperative guidelines prior to beginning the procedure.

TABLE 18.1 Recommended periods between discontinuation of the new anticoagulants and interventional pain procedure and the procedure and resumption of the new anticoagulant

Anticoagulant	Recommended period between discontinuation of drug and procedure*	Recommended interval between end of procedure and resumption of drug
Dabigatran	4–5 d	24 h
Dabigatran (renal disease)	6 d	24 h
Rivaroxaban	3 d	24 h
Apixaban	3–5 d**	24 h

* Conservative estimates of half-life were used given the lack of published studies and additional risks involved in patients with spine abnormalities.
** Longer intervals are recommended given the wide variability and potency of these drugs.
From reference 15.

Though there are no reports on the effect of aspirin on spine surgery, there is evidence that active aspirin use could be a risk factor for epidural hematoma, and low-dose aspirin use before spine surgery may lead to further blood drainage after surgery.[13-15] Non-aspirin nonsteroidal anti-inflammatory drugs (NSAIDs) can be discontinued without negatively affecting cardiac and cerebral function and thus can be effectively discontinued following 5 half-lives. COX-2 selective inhibitors do not need to be discontinued, as they do not have a significant impact on platelet function.[15] Patients taking fondaparinux and new oral anticoagulants (e.g., dabigatran, rivaroxaban, apixaban) should also follow this 5-half-life rule. If the risk of venous thromboembolism is determined to be unusually high by the treating physicians, new oral anticoagulants can be given at half the usual dose 12 hours after procedure completion.[15] Table 18.1 details the recommended duration sufficient for discontinuation of new anticoagulants.

There are anticoagulants that require shared decision-making to determine an appropriate plan for discontinuation prior to the procedure. Decisions about discontinuing phosphodiesterase inhibitors should be made among the interventionalist, the patient, and the prescribing physician. It is important to consider that dipyridamole, when combined with aspirin, has demonstrated an increased risk of bleeding.[16] Glycoprotein IIb/IIIa anticoagulants should also be reviewed by the involved physicians, as there is scant evidence available regarding the relationship between these medications and interventional procedures. Any patient who has recently received, or is recommended to receive, fibrinolytic agents should be referred to the managing service for additional review. Decisions regarding the cessation of P2Y12 inhibitors should also be made in conjunction with all treating physicians. Patients at high risk for bleeding typically meet one or more of the following criteria: concomitant use of anticoagulants, advanced age, presence of advanced liver or renal disease, and/or a history of abnormal bleeding. Table 18.2 details recommended intervals between discontinuation and resumption of P2Y12 inhibitors.

Table 18.3 details the recommended intervals between discontinuation and resumption of other common anticoagulants, including warfarin, heparin, and fondaparinux.

TABLE 18.2 Recommended periods between discontinuation of P2Y12 inhibitors and interventional pain procedure and between the procedure and resumption of P2Y12 inhibitors

Anticoagulant	Recommended period between discontinuation of drug and procedure*	Recommended interval between end of procedure and resumption of drug
Clopidogrel	7 d	12–24 h*
Prasugrel	7–10 d	24 h
Ticagrelor	5 d	24 h

* A typical daily dose (75 mg) can be started after 12 hours. If a loading dose is necessary, there should be a 24-hour interval after the procedure before resumption of clopidogrel.
From reference 15.

Patients taking warfarin who are considered to be at high risk for thrombosis may benefit from bridge therapy with low-molecular-weight heparin; however, this decision should be reviewed by all involved physicians.[15] Patients who are taking low-molecular-weight heparin should be handled with extreme caution when being reviewed for addition and/or resumption of concomitant drugs that affect hemostasis (antiplatelets, NSAIDs, selective serotonin reuptake inhibitors [SSRIs], and any other anticoagulants).[15]

There are also non-anticoagulant medications that should be reviewed and potentially discontinued prior to the procedure, as they have been associated with increased bleeding risk. Selective serotonin norepinephrine reuptake inhibitors (SNRIs) and SSRIs fall into this category and are associated with a heightened risk of bleeding when combined with concomitant anticoagulants, such as aspirin.[15] While routine discontinuation of SSRIs prior to the procedure is not recommended, patients who are determined to be at high risk by the

TABLE 18.3 Recommended period between discontinuation of anticoagulants and interventional pain procedure and between the procedure and resumption of anticoagulants

Anticoagulant	Recommended period between discontinuation of drug and procedure	Recommended interval between end of procedure and resumption of drug
Coumadin	5 d, normalization of INR	24 h
Intravenous heparin	4 h	2 h**
Subcutaneous heparin, BID and TID	8–10 h	2 h**
Low-molecular-weight heparin	24 h	24 h
Fibrinolytic agents	At least 48 h*	At least 48 h*
Fondaparinux	4 d	24 h

* Blood clots are not completely stable until approximately 10 days after fibrinolytic therapy. Increased bleeding may occur if procedure is conducted within 10 days of thrombolytic therapy.
** Increase to 24 hours if the procedure was especially bloody.
From reference 15.

treating physicians should be gradually tapered off their dosage of the medication. These medications follow the 5-half-life rule and tend to have long half-lives. Thus, tapering of these medications should begin weeks in advance of the procedure. SSRIs and SNRIs should be restarted as soon as possible once the risk of excessive bleeding dissipates, typically about 1 day after the procedure.[15]

Finally, there are some herbal and alternative therapies that may impact a patient's bleeding risk. Patients who are actively taking garlic and ginkgo biloba should be advised to stop taking them leading up to the procedure, and patients taking warfarin who are also taking dong quai, danshen, and/or Panax ginseng should receive similar instructions. While evidence on the weight of increased bleeding risk is limited, it is recommended that these remedies be discontinued in order to permit an ideal environment for the procedure.[15,17]

Risk of infection and complication

The patient's risk factors for postoperative infection need to be evaluated in the preoperative stage. Risk factors for developing an infection of the surgical site consist of smoking, diabetes, cancer, a weakened immune system, age, and being overweight. Generally, the risk of infection at the surgical site is higher in an open procedure than in a minimally invasive procedure, so this should be considered for patients undergoing open SIJ fusion surgery.

Administration of a preoperative antibiotic such as cefazolin is recommended for patients undergoing lumbar spine surgery in order to lower the risk of wound infection, urinary tract infection, or pneumonia.[18] This is something that should be done as a standard of care in patients undergoing SIJ fusion surgery. Patients undergoing either MIS or open SIJ fusion surgery should receive pre-incisional antibiotics.

A study on surgical site infection in spine surgery by Anderson et al. found the following information:

- Although not specific to SIJ fusion, a broad-spectrum antibiotic with specific coverage of *Staphylococcus aureus*, such as cephalosporin, is recommended as prophylaxis in most spine surgeries.
- Patients who are allergic to beta-lactam antibiotics should be given clindamycin.
- Avoidance of vancomycin is critical, given the risk of bacterial resistance, though the drug is effective in patients who test positive for MRSA.[19]

Administration of antibiotics within 30 minutes of surgery, as opposed to 30 to 60 minutes before surgery, has been shown to significantly decrease the risk of surgical site infection in cardiac surgery, hip/knee arthroplasty, and hysterectomy.[20] Preoperative warming may also decrease the risk of surgical site infection as well as the required number of antibiotic therapy courses postoperatively.[21] These findings should be further explored for SIJ fusion surgery specifically to lower the risk of postsurgical complications. Potential advantages of newer posterior-based approaches may include a lower incidence of perioperative complications due to the lower-profile technique and avoidance of neuraxial structures that can possibly occur with a lateral approach.

Setting expectations

Before surgery it is very important to make sure the patient understands the risks of the surgery as well as the potential for success. A literature review from 2015 found a mean patient "excellent satisfaction" rate of 84% for those who received MIS SIJ fusion surgery and 54% in those who received open SIJ fusion surgery.[22] Performing physicians need to discuss and be clear with their patients about the potential adverse events that can occur after undergoing SIJ fusion surgery. Some of the potential complications found in a retrospective comparative cohort study of patients who underwent SIJ fusion include bone fracture, buttock hematoma, cellulitis, deep venous thrombosis, facet pain, falls, hip pain, iliotibial band pain, leg pain, lipoma in wound scar requiring surgical removal, low back pain, pneumothorax, pulmonary embolism, and screw loosening.[12] An overall postoperative adverse event rate of 18% in patients who underwent an MIS approach and 21% in patients who underwent an open approach has been reported.[12]

Conclusion

To obtain the best outcomes in SIJ fusion surgery, preoperative considerations are of major importance, specifically patient comorbidities, the type of SIJ fusion performed, anticoagulation, risk of infection, and preoperative physical exam.

References

1. Schwarzer AC, Aprill CN, Bogduk N. The sacroiliac joint in chronic low back pain. *Spine*. 1995;20:31–37.
2. Raj MA, Ampat G, Varacallo M. Sacroiliac joint pain. StatPearls. https://www.ncbi.nlm.nih.gov/books/NBK470299/
3. Bernard TN Jr, Kirkaldy-Willis WH. Recognizing specific characteristics of nonspecific low back pain. *Clin Orthop Relat Res*. 1987;217:266–280.
4. Sembrano JN, Polly DW Jr. How often is low back pain not coming from the back? *Spine*. 2009;34(1):E27–E32. doi:10.1097/BRS.0b013e31818b8882. PMID: 19127145.
5. Whang P, Cher D, Polly D, et al. Sacroiliac joint fusion using triangular titanium implants vs. nonsurgical management: Six-month outcomes from a prospective randomized controlled trial. *Int J Spine Surg*. 2015;9:6. doi:10.14444/2006
6. INSITE Study Group. Randomized controlled trial of minimally invasive sacroiliac joint fusion using triangular titanium implants vs. nonsurgical management for sacroiliac joint dysfunction: 12-month outcomes. *Neurosurgery*. 2015;77(5):674–691. doi:10.1227/NEU.0000000000000988
7. Szadek KM, van der Wurff P, van Tulder MW, et al. Diagnostic validity of criteria for sacroiliac joint pain: A systematic review. *J Pain*. 2009;10(4):354–368. doi:10.1016/j.jpain.2008.09.014. PMID: 19101212.
8. Dydyk AM, Forro SD, Hanna A. Sacroiliac joint injury. StatPearls. https://www.ncbi.nlm.nih.gov/books/NBK557881/

9. Narouze S, Benzon HT, Provenzano D, et al. Interventional spine and pain procedures in patients on antiplatelet and anticoagulant medications (second edition): Guidelines from the American Society of Regional Anesthesia and Pain Medicine, the European Society of Regional Anaesthesia and Pain Therapy, the American Academy of Pain Medicine, the International Neuromodulation Society, the North American Neuromodulation Society, and the World Institute of Pain. *Reg Anesth Pain Med.* 2018;43(3):225–262. doi:10.1097/AAP.0000000000000700. PMID: 29278603.

10. Ledonio CGT, Polly DW, Swiontkowski MF. Minimally invasive versus open sacroiliac joint fusion: Are they similarly safe and effective? *Clin Orthop Rel Res.* 2014;472(6):1831–1838.

11. Yson SC, Sembrano JN, Polly Jr DW. Sacroiliac joint fusion: Approaches and recent outcomes. *PM&R.* 2019;11:S114–S117.

12. Smith AG, Capobianco R, Cher D, et al. Open versus minimally invasive sacroiliac joint fusion: A multi-center comparison of perioperative measures and clinical outcomes. *Ann Surg Innov Res.* 2013;7(1):14. doi:10.1186/1750-1164-7-14. PMID: 24172188; PMCID: PMC3817574.

13. Kang S-B, Cho K-J, Moon K-H, et al. Does low-dose aspirin increase blood loss after spinal fusion surgery? *Spine J.* 2011;11(4):303–307.

14. Kou J, Fischgrund J, Biddinger A., Herkowitz H. Risk factors for spinal epidural hematoma after spinal surgery. *Spine.* 2002;27(15):1670–1673.

15. Narouze S, Benzon HT, Provenzano DA, et al. Interventional spine and pain procedures in patients on antiplatelet and anticoagulant medications: Guidelines from the American Society of Regional Anesthesia and Pain Medicine, the European Society of Regional Anaesthesia and Pain Therapy, the American Academy of Pain Medicine, the International Neuromodulation Society, the North American Neuromodulation Society, and the World Institute of Pain. *Reg Anesth Pain Med.* 2015;40(3):182–212.

16. Hall R, Mazer CD. Antiplatelet drugs: A review of their pharmacology and management in the perioperative period. *Anesth Analg.* 2011;112(2):292–318.

17. Horlocker TT, Wedel DJ, Rowlingson JC, et al. Regional anesthesia in the patient receiving antithrombotic therapy or thrombolytic therapy: American Society of Regional Anesthesia and Pain Medicine evidence-based guidelines (third edition). *Reg Anesth Pain Med.* 2010;35:64–101.

18. Rubinstein E, Findler G, Amit P, Shaked I. Perioperative prophylactic cephazolin in spinal surgery. A double-blind placebo-controlled trial. *J Bone Joint Surg Br.* 1994;76(1):99–102. PMID: 8300691.

19. Anderson PA, Savage JW, Vaccaro AR, et al. Prevention of surgical site infection in spine surgery. *Neurosurgery.* 2017;80(3S):S114–S123.

20. Steinberg J, Braun BI, Hellinger WC, et al. Timing of antimicrobial prophylaxis and the risk of surgical site infections: Results from the Trial to Reduce Antimicrobial Prophylaxis Errors. *Ann Surg.* 2009;250(1):10–16.

21. Melling AC, Ali B, Scott EM, Leaper DJ. Effects of preoperative warming on the incidence of wound infection after clean surgery: A randomised controlled trial. *Lancet.* 2001;358(9285):876–880.

22. Zaidi HA, Montoure AJ, Dickman CA. Surgical and clinical efficacy of sacroiliac joint fusion: A systematic review of the literature. *J Neurosurg Spine.* 2015;23(1):59–66.

19

Lateral fusion

Gustaf Van Acker, Jonathon Belding, and
Chong H. Kim

Introduction

Sacroiliac joint (SIJ) fusion is a procedure for treating chronic low back pain due to sacroiliac dysfunction and sacroiliitis that has been approved by the U.S. Food and Drug Administration (FDA). According to a market analysis, it is estimated that the global minimally invasive surgical (MIS) SIJ fusion market will reach $450 million by the end of 2025.[1] In 2017, the United States and Europe accounted for 85% of this sizable and rapidly growing market.

Yet prior to 2008, surgical fixation was relatively scarce. This dramatic shift is the result of multiple factors, including the change in surgical approach from open to MIS. SIJ fusion was introduced by Smith-Petersen in 1921 when he developed an open posterolateral transiliac approach.[2] This Smith-Petersen approach remained the standard in SIJ fusion, with slight improvements and modifications over time.[3,4] However, open surgery had the typical complications of blood loss, tissue stripping, and a long and painful recovery time.[5] In 2008, two groups introduced percutaneous approaches to SIJ fusion: Wise and Dall introduced a percutaneous posterior approach[6] and Al-Khayer et al. introduced the percutaneous lateral approach.[7] That same year the FDA granted 510(k) approval for the first lateral percutaneous system, the iFuse Implant System by SI Bone (510(k) is a premarket submission made to the FDA to demonstrate that a device to be marketed is as safe and effective [or substantially equivalent] to a legally marketed device). By 2012, 85% of SIJ fusions were being performed using the MIS technique.[6]

Concurrently, the SIJ joint has become increasingly implicated as the cause of refractory back pain in as many as 30% of those with back complaints.[8] The conjunction of increasing SIJ dysfunction diagnosis, reimbursement policy changes, and technique improvement has resulted in the burgeoning of the procedure as well as the number of companies manufacturing MIS SIJ fusion systems: As of this writing there are over 25 FDA-approved SIJ fusion systems on the market, at least 14 of which are designed for a lateral approach (Box 19.1).

BOX 19.1. FDA-approved MIS SIJ fusion systems for lateral approach

Blue Topaz™ CompresSIve Sacroiliac Screw System, Osseus

Entasis® Sacroiliac Joint Fusion System, CoreLink LLC

EVOL®SI system, Cutting Edge Spine®

Sacroiliac Joint Fusion System, Genesys Spine®

iFuse Implant System®, SI Bone®

M.U.S.T. ® Sacro Iliac Screws System, Medacta International

SambaScrew®, Orthofix®

Siconus™, Camber Spine

SiCure™ Sacroiliac Fusion System, Alevio®

Silex® Sacroiliac Joint Fusion System, XTANT Medical

SI-LOK® Sacroiliac Joint Fixation System, Globus® Medical

SImmetry®, RTI Surgical®

SImpact™, LifeSpine®

TriCor™, Zimmer Biomet Spine, Inc.

Multiple approaches now exist to fuse the SIJ, the most common being MIS lateral and MIS posterior approaches. Some systems apply a combination of MIS lateral and posterior approaches. Both open posterior and open Smith-Petersen posterolateral transiliac approaches may also still be used in cases where the MIS technique is not an option. There are alternative approaches being developed as well, such as the oblique lateral approach and mini-open combined with MIS.[8,9] This chapter will detail the lateral approaches to SIJ arthrodesis.

Implant devices

Materials for lateral SIJ fusion vary among companies, with many involving proprietary properties of surface treatment, coatings, and thread design (Figure 19.1). However, most implants incorporate the following properties, all of which are aimed at inducing osseointegration, enhancing and maintaining arthrodesis, and decreasing the chances of hardware loosening:

1. A cannulated shaft for navigating the implants over a guide wire. Some screw implants are self-tapping, obviating the need to drill a pilot hole. By designing and manufacturing all of the tools and implants with cannulation that interfaces with a guide wire, the accuracy of the trajectory and final placement of the implants is enhanced.

2. Slots or fenestrations for incorporating autograft, allograft (cadaver), or synthetic bone graft. Synthetic bone graft is composed of hydroxyapatite $[Ca_{10}(PO_4)_6(OH)_2]$, calcium

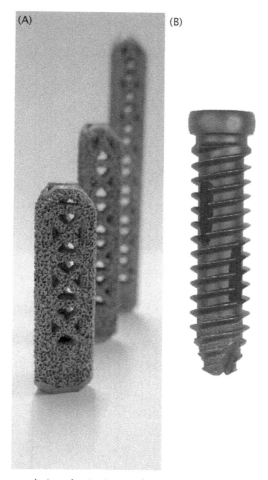

FIGURE 19.1. (**A**) Fenestrated triangular titanium implants printed with a surface that mimics trabecular cancellous bone. (**B**) Slotted, hydroxyapatite-coated and SintrOS™ laser surface-treated screws. *Source:* **A**, printed with permission from iFuse-3D™, SI Bone®. **B**, printed with permission from SI-LOK® Sacroiliac Joint Fixation System, Globus® Medical.

sulfates, calcium phosphates, or other osteoconductive biomaterials.[10] Some devices, such as Entasis by CoreLink LLC, are designed to both produce and place autograft into the joint concurrent with the insertion of the screw implants, thereby reducing the number of steps in incorporating graft into the implant/joint interface. The fenestrations also allow ingrowth and through-growth of remodeling bone, enhancing intraarticular fusion.

3. Micro- and nano-level surface preparation that creates a microenvironment similar to native bone. The goal of this is to encourage on-growth of native bone to the implant.

4. Some form of hydroxyapatite or other osteoconductive biomaterial adhered to the implant surface to encourage on-growth of bone to the implant.

Implants have been typically machined out of medical-grade titanium alloy. More recently, additive manufacturing (three-dimensional printing) is being explored in the medical implant manufacturing process. Porous titanium scaffolding created through 3D printing allows for creation of complex implant shapes and surface textures that may enhance biocompatibility and may optimize bone ingrowth.[11] In 2017 the FDA approved the first SIJ fusion implant printed from titanium, iFuse-3D.

Lateral SIJ arthrodesis
SIJ fusion performed using fluoroscopic guidance

The MIS lateral approach to SIJ fusion may be performed using fluoroscopic guidance. Image guidance is necessary to plan trajectories and ensure correct placement of instrumentation while minimizing the risk of adjacent nerve and soft tissue damage.

This procedure is typically conducted under general anesthesia, although it may be performed under monitored anesthesia care (MAC) anesthesia. The patient is placed in the prone position on a flat-topped radiolucent surgical table appropriate for spine surgery, such as a Jackson table and Wilson supporting frame (OSI, Union City, CA, USA).[12,13] Due to the risk of neurologic damage of L5, S1, and S2 nerve roots, intraoperative neurophysiology monitoring (IONM) may be performed. Electrodes can be placed on the anterior tibialis, the gastrocnemius, and the rectal sphincter to monitor L5, S1, and S2 nerve roots, respectively.[14] The patient's skin is sterilized and the patient is draped in the usual fashion, leaving the target hip exposed. A C-arm image scanner intensifier is used to obtain lateral, inlet, outlet, and true anteroposterior (AP) views of the SIJ. A true AP view should be perpendicular to the dorsal SIJ line. For the lateral view, true lateral is ensured by aligning the sacral notches and alae. Skin points overlying the ala and the dorsal SIJ line are marked to their convergence, which is the rostrodorsal edge of the SIJ. At this point the procedure may be performed percutaneously for each implant, or one incision may be performed for all implants. An approximately 3-cm incision is made at or just dorsal to the dorsal sacral line and just caudal to the ala line (Figure 19.2). A guide wire is inserted so that the tip is at the dorsal edge of the sacral joint when the tip meets the ilium. Viewing in true AP, the guide wire is driven through the SIJ sacrum using a surgical mallet while aiming for the S1 pedicle, stopping lateral to the neural foramen (Figure 19.3A). Image guidance is performed to ensure the tip of the guide wire remains stable throughout the procedure.

Dilating cannulas with increasing diameter are inserted until reaching desired dilation, while ensuring the dilators are flush with the ilium. Leaving the outer dilating cannula in place, a depth gauge is inserted over the guide wire until it meets the lateral wall of the ilium, and the length of the first screw to be implanted is determined. The depth gauge is removed. A cannulated drill bit is inserted into a standard high-speed surgical drill and the drill bit is guided onto the guide wire. A pilot hole is then drilled to a depth just distal to the joint cortices. After the drill bit is removed, a cannulated screw is attached to an associated screwdriver. Depending on the system used, the screw may be loaded with autograft, allograft (cadaver), or synthetic bone graft. The screw and driver are slid over the

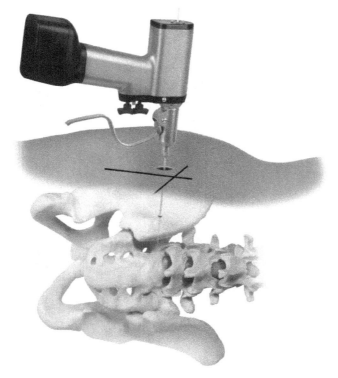

FIGURE 19.2. Image illustrating insertion of a guide wire through the left SIJ. The skin is marked delineating the dorsal wall of the sacrum intersecting with the sacral ala. An incision is made dorsal to the posterior wall of the sacrum and caudal to the edge of the ala. A guide wire is advanced to the lateral ilium and advanced with a drill through the SI joint but lateral to the neural foramen. *Source:* Printed with permission from SI-LOK® Sacroiliac Joint Fixation System, Globus® Medical.

guide wire and, once at bone, are screwed clockwise until the screw head is flush with bone. Fluoroscopy is used to monitor and ensure appropriate screw trajectory. The driver is detached from the screw and removed while retaining the guide wire. The first screw is now in place (Figure 19.3B), and the dilating cannula is removed.

Two or three screws are required for sufficient arthrodesis. For placement of the second screw, most systems have an alignment guide that slides over the first guide wire and provides guided placement of the second caudal guide wire placement. After placement of the second guide wire, the first guide wire and alignment guide may be removed. The steps used for the first screw placement are then applied for the second screw (Figure 19.3C). This process may be done for a third and final screw. The three screws should be relatively equally spaced and parallel to one another (Figure 19.3D).

After the implants are in place, instrumentation is removed and hemostasis is applied. Layered closure is performed sequentially, and a compressive dressing is applied. This MIS procedure takes approximately 1 hour to perform. Benefits to using an MIS approach over an open approach are reduced blood loss, decreased chance of soft tissue stripping, smaller incision, shorter hospital length of stay, reduced pain, and shorter recovery time.[15]

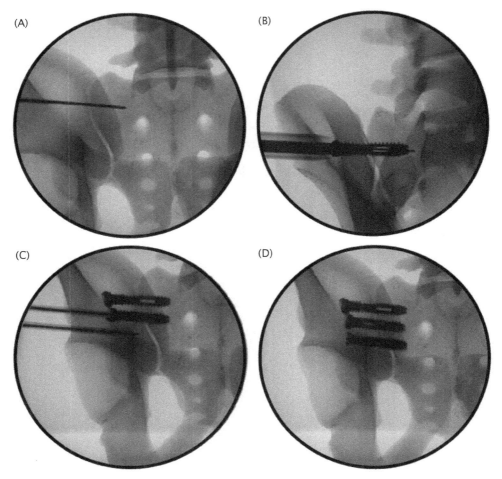

FIGURE 19.3. AP fluoroscopic images of a left lateral MIS SIJ fusion. (**A**) A guide wire is advanced through the SIJ but lateral to the neural foramen. (**B**) First implant is advanced through soft tissue dilator and screwed into place over the guide wire. (**C**) With the first screw in place, the second and third screws are placed using an alignment guide. (**D**) Three screws are in place, and implantation is complete. *Source:* Printed with permission from SI-LOK® Sacroiliac Joint Fixation System, Globus® Medical.

SIJ fusion performed using a navigation system

The MIS lateral approach to SIJ fusion may be performed using a navigation system, such as excelsiusGPS, NAV3i (Stryker), or Medtronic StealthStation, in conjunction with navigation instruments, such as iFuse-Navigation. A navigation system allows the surgeon to visualize where instrumentation is relative to anatomic location in real time by overlaying navigation instruments on intraoperative CT imaging, such as O-arm (Medtronic) or Airo (Brainlab).

This procedure is conducted under general anesthesia. The patient is placed in the prone position on a radiolucent flat-topped surgical table such as a Jackson table and Wilson supporting frame.[13] As discussed in the previous section, due to the risk of neurologic damage of L5, S1, and S2 nerve roots, IONM may be performed. Electrodes can be placed on the anterior tibialis, the gastrocnemius, and the rectal sphincter for L5, S1, and S2 nerve roots, respectively.[14] The navigation system camera is positioned at the foot of the table with a good line of sight to the patient's pelvis. The navigation system monitor should be placed so that the surgeon can readily refer to the navigation imaging while performing the procedure. A navigation frame may be placed on the ipsilateral or contralateral side. Palpate for the posterior superior iliac spine (PSIS), where the guide pin will be placed. The patient's skin is sterilized and the patient is draped in the usual fashion, leaving the target hip exposed. The skin is marked, and a stab incision is made overlying the PSIS. A navigating radiopaque disposable percutaneous pin of appropriate length is inserted through the incision to the SIJ, and the pin is impacted into place through the SIJ using a surgical mallet. A navigation frame is then placed on the exposed pin with reflective marker spheres facing the navigation camera. Prior to introducing the mobile intraoperative CT into place, it is optional to cover the navigation frame with a transparent drape to protect the sterility of the frame while allowing the camera to detect the reflective spheres. The CT is positioned over the SIJ, and AP and lateral scout images are obtained to ensure the CT is positioned correctly in rostral–caudal and ventral–dorsal planes. To help limit motion artifact during image capture, the anesthesiologist may momentarily suspend the patient's breathing. Navigation tools, or tools with reflective spheres on them, are independently placed on the navigation reference frame to register with the system.

The planar navigation probe is used to demarcate the planned incision lines on the exposed hip. The planned rostral implant is identified using the planar probe, and the SIJ is demarcated from rostral to caudal. The skin then is marked for incision overlying the length of the SIJ. At this point the procedure may be performed percutaneously for each implant, or one incision may be performed for all implants. A skin incision is made, and the planar probe shaft is inserted to the lateral ilium at the rostral end of the SIJ. This provides information on planned trajectory and depth. After removing the planar probe, a navigation drill guide is advanced along the same trajectory to the lateral ilium. A digital projection from the tip of the drill guide projecting through the SIJ can inform the length of screw that will eventually be placed through the SIJ. A guide wire is then advanced through the drill guide until it meets the ilium. Once in place, a power drill is connected to the guide wire, and the wire is advanced to the appropriate depth as determined using navigation. The drill guide and drill are removed while retaining the guide wire in place. A blunt dissector is fed over the guide wire to dissect gluteal muscle, after which the dissector is removed. A soft tissue protector is then placed over the guide wire to help ensure there is no damage to at-risk structures. Once abutted to the lateral ilium, the internal canula is removed and a cannulated drill is fed onto the guide wire until meeting with the ilium. A hole is drilled into the lateral ilium and then the drill is removed. Next, a navigating broach is fed over the guide wire and hammered into place so that the broach head enters the sacrum. While securing the guide wire to minimize movement, the broach is hammered out and off of the wire.

The implant of appropriate size is chosen, and optional grafting material is placed into implant fenestrations. The implant is fed onto the guide wire and either screwed into place or hammered using an impactor, depending on the device. This process is repeated once or

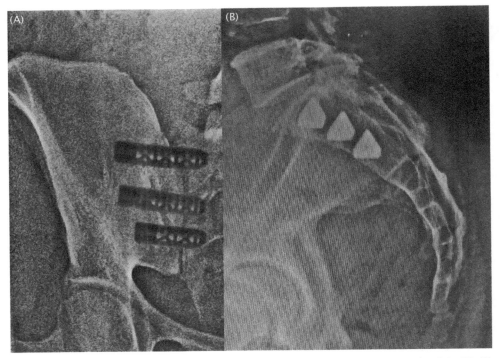

FIGURE 19.4. (**A**) AP pelvis x-ray showing radiopaque triangular implants spanning the right SIJ. (**B**) Lateral view showing the three implants spanning the SIJ from rostral to caudal. *Source:* Printed with permission from iFuse-3D™, SI Bone®.

twice using an adjustable guide placed over the first guide wire for a total of two or three implants. The caudal implant can be aimed toward the body of S2. After implants are in place, all instrumentation is removed and hemostasis is performed. Layered closure is performed sequentially, and a compressive dressing is applied. Figure 19.4 shows AP and lateral films of the implants in place.

SIJ fusion performed using an open approach

SIJ arthrodesis can be achieved using a posterior lateral open technique modified from that pioneered by Smith-Petersen in 1921.[2] While hardware and surgical techniques have improved since that time, which has improved safety and efficacy, the general approach remains the same.[3] Using a transiliac approach allows the surgeon to avoid the posterior ligamentous complex of the SIJ.

This procedure is conducted under general anesthesia. The patient is placed in the prone position on a radiolucent flat-topped surgical table such as a Jackson table and Wilson supporting frame.[13] The patient's skin is sterilized and the patient is draped in the usual fashion, leaving the target hip exposed. Presurgical CT imaging can give information about anatomy and measurements intraoperatively.[16] Fluoroscopic identification of the PSIS is made, and the skin is marked overlying the iliac crest. An 8- to 10-cm curvilinear incision is made along the crest, and electrocautery is used to dissect to the fascial attachment at the iliac crest. Subperiosteal dissection is performed until the posterior and lateral aspects of the ilium surface are exposed. Measurements from CT imaging can help provide the anatomic location of the ilium, as well as the expected ilium thickness at this level, which may be 15 to 20 mm or greater.[16] The boundaries of the sacrum in apposition with the ilium are within the boundaries of the sciatic notch and the anterior gluteal line. At this time cancellous screws may be placed in the rostral and caudal ends of the SIJ,[16] or a plate and screws may be used to stabilize the joint at the end of the procedure.[3] A rectangular window is made through the ilium exposing the articular surface of the sacral side of the joint and is removed en bloc. The articular cartilage and the subchondral bone are curetted from both the bone block and the sacral side of the joint, and the bone block is reinserted. Corticocancellous PSIS bone autograft may be packed into the window prior to block insertion. The block is countersunk, allowing for apposition of cancellous surfaces of the bone block and joint. The joint is stabilized with a plate and screws.[3] Muscle and fascia are approximated and closed with absorbable sutures, a subcutaneous drain is placed, and superficial closure is performed. The patients are toe touch weight bearing for 6 to 12 weeks until evidence of fusion is observed.[3,16]

Safety

Lateral MIS SIJ fusion has been shown to have an improved safety profile compared to the posterior lateral open approach, with lower surgical complication rates and lower rates of nonunion.[3,8,15,17,18] Open fusion complications include increased rates of blood loss during surgery, pseudoarthrosis, deep wound infection, and painful hardware. With a lateral MIS approach there is a risk of injuring or impinging on the sacral nerve roots as they exit their neural foramen, as well as roots within the canal itself. Care must be taken to stay lateral to the neural foramen to avoid this and to employ imaging and IONM when placing hardware.

Postsurgical complications are reported in MIS cases. A retrospective study by Schoell et al. in 2016 reported a 16.4% complication rate and new lumbar pathology at 6-month postoperative follow-up (men, 9.1%; women, ≤3.3%).[19] Duhon et al. in 2013 performed a 6-month prospective study using the iFuse Implant System, and 52 adverse events occurred in 34 of the 94 subjects by the end of the 6-month follow-up period.[20] Most of the events were nonemergent, such as hip, back, and buttock pain; six events were rated as severe, with two being probably or definitely related to the procedure. Ledonio et al. in 2014 performed a retrospective single-site study comparing the safety and efficacy of MIS versus open fusion; they showed higher estimated blood loss, a longer surgical time, and a longer hospital stay in the patient undergoing open fusion compared to those undergoing MIS.[21]

Shamrock et al. in 2019 performed a systematic review of existing literature to assess the safety profile of MIS SIJ fusion.[22] Fourteen studies were included. Their findings revealed an 11.1% complication rate, with the most common complication being surgical wound infection/drainage (n = 17/819 joints, 2%). Three percent of complications involved the implant itself, with nerve root impingement being the most common issue (n = 13/819, 1.6%). They concluded that while the procedure is relatively safe, it is not without certain complications. They recommend improvements in patient optimization and surgical technique and suggest the use of real-time intraoperative imaging.

Efficacy

Lateral SIJ fusion has shown good efficacy in both open and MIS cases, although recent studies suggest better outcomes with MIS procedures. Smith et al. in 2013 conducted a multi-center, retrospective comparative cohort study comparing open to MIS approach. Mean visual analog scale (VAS) change from baseline at 24 months was −5.6 and −2.0 for MIS and open SIJ fusion, respectively.[15] In addition, the study revealed significantly less estimated blood loss during surgery (33 vs. 288 cc) as well as decreased operating time (70 vs. 163 minutes) and hospital stay (1.3 vs. 5.1 days) in the MIS group compared to the open group. Of note, in this study 44% of the open surgery patients underwent explanation, primarily due to pain at screw sites. This is significantly higher than the 3.5% of MIS patients who eventually underwent repositioning due to nerve root impingement.

Other studies have reported similar success using the same implant and approach as the Smith et al. (2013) study (Table 19.1). In 2012 Rudolf reported a VAS improvement of −4.3 at 12 months, with an 82% patient satisfaction rate.[23] These results extended to 5 years, at which point there was a sustained VAS improvement of −5.9 from the presurgical baseline 5 years prior, and satisfaction was maintained at 82%.[24] Sachs et al. in 2012 showed a −6.2 VAS improvement at 12 months,[25] and Cummings et al. in 2013 showed a −6.6 VAS improvement at 12 months.[26] Data from Duhon et al. (2016) revealed that at the 2-year follow-up after MIS SIJ fusion, patients had sustained improvement in VAS (−5.4 from baseline) as well as improvements in the Oswestry Disability Index (ODI) score and quality of life.[27] Patel et al. in 2019 found a −5.1 VAS improvement and a 23.6-point improvement in the ODI at 6 months.[28] Other studies have reported similar findings, with good improvement in pain scores, disability scores, and fusion.[7,29]

Studies investigating MIS SIJ fusion report primarily on back pain; however, some report pain relief in the legs with significant results. Kube et al.[33] in 2016 reported that, at 12 months follow-up, back pain improved from 81.7 to 44.1 points ($p < .001$) and leg pain from 63.6 to 27.7 points ($p = .001$). Rappoport et al.[46] in 2017 reported that, at 12 months follow-up, VAS for back pain improved from 55.8 ± 26.7 mm preoperatively to 32.7 ± 27.4 mm postoperatively ($p < .01$) and VAS for leg pain improved from 40.6 ± 29.5 mm to 12.5 ± 23.3 mm.

A 5-year prospective study by Whang et al. in 2019 reported an improvement of −54 on the 100-point VAS and an ODI decrease of 26 points.[30] Heiney et al. in 2015 performed a systematic review and meta-analysis of lateral approach MIS clinical outcomes. The study revealed a mean surgical time of 59 minutes, estimated blood loss 36.9 cc, 1.7 days for hospital length of stay, an ODI decrease of 31 points by 12 months, and a −6.1 VAS improvement at 24 months.[31] They concluded that studies consistently report rapid, sustained, and clinically important improvements in SIJ pain, disability, and quality-of-life scores.

TABLE 19.1 Current evidence for lateral approach for MIS SIJ fusion

Author, year	Implant	Patients (#)	Follow-up (months)	ΔVAS/NRS	ΔODI	Fusion (%)	Notes
Al-Khayer et al., 2008[7]	HMA screw	9	24	−3.5	−14		
Khurana et al., 2009[29]	HMA screw	15	9–39				SF-36 improved from 37 to 80
Rudolf, 2012[23]	iFuse	50	12	−4.9			71% clinically significant improvement
Sachs et al., 2012[25]	iFuse	11	12	−6.2			82% patient satisfaction
Smith et al., 2013[15]	iFuse	114	12	−6.2			
Cummings et al., 2013[26]	iFuse	18	12	−6.6	−37.5		95% patient satisfaction
Rudolf et al., 2013[37]	iFuse	40	24	−5.8/ −5.47			Patients with prior lumbar fusion or no fusion
Sachs et al., 2013[38]	iFuse	40	12	−7.8			
Gaetani et al., 2013[39]	iFuse	10	8–18	−4.0	−19.4		
Duhon et al., 2013[20]	iFuse	94	6	−4.9	−15.8		
Mason et al., 2013[40]	HMA screw	55	12–84	−3.5			Included patients from Khurana et al., 2009[29]
Rudolf et al., 2014[24]	iFuse	17	60	−5.9		87	88% clinically significant improvement
Schroeder et al., 2014[41]	iFuse	6	10	−5.2	−11.7		
Sachs et al., 2014[42]	iFuse	144	12	−6.1			Includes 18 patients from Cummings et al.[26] & 40 from Sachs et al.[38]
Sachs et al., 2016[43]	iFuse	107		−4.8			Includes patients from Sachs et al., 2014[42]
Duhon et al., 2016[27]	iFuse	172	24	−5.4	−24.3		Prospective MC
Kube et al., 2016[33]	SImmetry	20	12	−3.8	−20.5	88	

(continued)

TABLE 19.1   Continued

Author, year	Implant	Patients (#)	Follow-up (months)	ΔVAS/NRS	ΔODI	Fusion (%)	Notes
Polly et al., 2016[44]	iFuse	102	24	−5.5	−28.4		SIJ fusion vs. conservative, Level 1 prospective
Kancherla et al., 2017[45]	iFuse SambaScrew	36 9					Only postop VAS and ODI
Rappoport et al., 2017[46]	SI-LOK	32	12	−2.3			
Araghi et al., 2017[47]	SI-LOK	50	6	−4.1	−20.2		
Dengler et al., 2017[48]	iFuse	52	12	−4.2	−25.0		Level 1 prospective
Cross et al., 2018[32]	SImmetry	19	24			79	94% satisfaction rate
Darr et al., 2018[49]	iFuse	103	36	−5.5	−28.2		Prospective MC, 82% very satisfied
Patel et al., 2019[28]	iFuse	28	6	−5.1	−23.6		Prospective MC
Whang et al., 2019[30]	iFuse	103	60	−5.4	−26	87	Prospective MC
Claus et al., 2020[50]	iFuse	82	12	−2.4			

Visual analog scale (VAS) and numeric rating scale (NRS) for reported back pain are provided on a 10-point scale, and Oswestry Disability Index (ODI) is based on a 100-point scale. HMA: hollow modular anchorage; MC: multi-center.

A systematic review of available manuscripts on MIS SIJ fusion by Shamrock et al. in 2019 revealed a mean VAS improvement of −5.3 and an ODI improvement of 28.0.[22]

Rates of successful fusion have increased with newer technology and MIS lateral SIJ fusion techniques. Fusion rates are not always reported, but when they are, successful fusion rates range from 25% to 90%.[24,27,32,33] With open SIJ fusions, the rate of pseudoarthrosis, or non-union, has been reported to be 41.2%.[17] Smith et al. in 2013 compared open SIJ fusion to MIS SIJ fusion and found pseudoarthrosis, screw loosening, and implant irritation were sources of surgical revision in 43% of patients. The MIS group had none of these complications.[15] However, in 2005, Buchowski et al. used a modified Smith-Petersen technique with the addition of a T- or L-shaped plate and screws spanning the joint and 12-week non-weight-bearing status and reported that 85% of patients achieved solid fusion.[3] Whang et al. in 2019 reported an 88% joint fusion rate, evidenced through CT imaging, at 5 years after implantation.[30]

In 2020 Martin et al. published a solid review of the current literature for lateral MIS SIJ fusion.[34] In it they provide a pooled analysis of all existing data, showing a mean decrease of 80.3 to 32.2 (100-point scale) in VAS and a mean decrease of 56.2 to 34.4 in ODI. They conclude that MIS SIJF provides significant improvement in pain scores and disability in most patients.

One limitation in the data is that the majority of evidence reported has been retrospective. Also, while there are many device manufacturers, the majority of studies published were conducted with the iFuse Implant System (SI Bone). The field would benefit from Level 1 prospective studies and studies involving other SIJ fusion systems on the market.

One hypothetical concern for SIJ fusion is adjacent joint dysfunction resulting from the fusion. However, there is no significant evidence to date that this occurs. Using an experimentally validated finite element model, Lindsey et al. in 2015 suggested that SIJ fusion using triangular titanium implants results in minimal change in range of motion of the lumbar spine.[35] Similarly, Joukar et al. in 2019 applied the same model to assess change in stress at the hip joint following SIJ fusion and found no significant change, suggesting that adjacent segment disease is likely low.[36] Future clinical studies aimed at assessing adjacent segment disease following MIS SIJ fusion are warranted.

Conclusion

Lateral sacroiliac arthrodesis is rapidly becoming a frequently performed procedure in patients with SIJ pain. SIJ dysfunction is implicated as the pain generator in up to 30% of patients with back pain complaints. The emergence of percutaneous approaches for SIJ fusion has improved many safety and efficacy outcome measures in comparison to traditional open approaches. However, when MIS technique is not feasible, an open posterolateral approach remains a relatively safe and effective option for refractory SIJ pain.

References

1. 360 Market Updates. Global MIS sacroiliac joint fusion market insights, forecast to 2025. https://www.360marketupdates.com/global-mis-sacroiliac-joint-fusion-market-13716161
2. Smith-Petersen, M. N. Arthrodesis of the sacroiliac joint. A new method of approach. *J Bone Joint Surg Am* **3**, 400–405 (1921).
3. Buchowski, J. M., *et al.* Functional and radiographic outcome of sacroiliac arthrodesis for the disorders of the sacroiliac joint. *Spine J* **5**, 520–529, doi:10.1016/j.spinee.2005.02.022 (2005).
4. Smith-Petersen, M. N., & Rogers, WA. End-result study of arthrodesis of the sacroiliac joint for arthritis—traumatic and nontraumatic. *J Bone Joint Surg Am* **8**, 118–136 (1926).
5. Lorio, M. P., *et al.* Utilization of minimally invasive surgical approach for sacroiliac joint fusion in surgeon population of ISASS and SMISS membership. *Open Orthop J* **8**, 1–6, doi:10.2174/1874325001408010001 (2014).
6. International Society for the Advancement of Spinal Surgery. Statement on coding changes for minimally invasive SI joint fusion. http://www.isass.org/public_policy/2013-08-07-isass-statement-minimally-invasive-si-joint-fusion-coding-changes.html
7. Al-Khayer, A., *et al.* Percutaneous sacroiliac joint arthrodesis: A novel technique. *J Spinal Disord Tech* **21**, 359–363, doi:10.1097/BSD.0b013e318145ab96 (2008).
8. Cleveland, A. W., 3rd, *et al.* Mini-open sacroiliac joint fusion with direct bone grafting and minimally invasive fixation using intraoperative navigation. *J Spine Surg* **5**, 31–37, doi:10.21037/jss.2019.01.04 (2019).
9. Dube-Cyr, R., *et al.* Biomechanical analysis of two insertion sites for the fixation of the sacroiliac joint via an oblique lateral approach. *Clin Biomech* **74**, 118–123, doi:10.1016/j.clinbiomech.2020.02.010 (2020).
10. Choi, J., *et al.* The role of orthobiologics in orthopaedics. In *Biologics in orthopaedic surgery* (eds. A. D. Mazzocca & A. D. Lindsay), Chapter 1, pp. 1–8 (2019). Elsevier.

11. Sidambe, A. T. Biocompatibility of advanced manufactured titanium implants: A review. *Materials* **7**, 8168–8188, doi:10.3390/ma7128168 (2014).

12. Globus Medical. SI-LOK Select sacroiliac joint fusion system surgical technique guide.

13. Schonauer, C., *et al.* Positioning on surgical table. *Eur Spine J* **13**(Suppl 1), S50–S55, doi:10.1007/s00586-004-0728-y (2004).

14. iFuse surgical technique. https://si-bone.com/providers/solutions/ifuse-assisting-technologies/ifuse-neuromonitoring-kit

15. Smith, A. G., *et al.* Open versus minimally invasive sacroiliac joint fusion: A multi-center comparison of perioperative measures and clinical outcomes. *Ann Surg Innov Res* **7**, 14, doi:10.1186/1750-1164-7-14 (2013).

16. Moore, M. R. Posterior lateral open approach for sacroiliac joint arthrodesis. In *Surgery for the painful, dysfunctional sacroiliac joint* (eds. B. E. Dall *et al.*), Chapter 11, 119–132 (2015). Springer.

17. Schutz, U., & Grob, D. Poor outcome following bilateral sacroiliac joint fusion for degenerative sacroiliac joint syndrome. *Acta Orthop Belg* **72**, 296–308 (2006).

18. Ashman, B., *et al.* Chronic sacroiliac joint pain: Fusion versus denervation as treatment options. *Evid Based Spine Care J* **1**, 35–44, doi:10.1055/s-0030-1267066 (2010).

19. Schoell, K., *et al.* Postoperative complications in patients undergoing minimally invasive sacroiliac fusion. *Spine J* **16**, 1324–1332, doi:10.1016/j.spinee.2016.06.016 (2016).

20. Duhon, B. S., *et al.* Safety and 6-month effectiveness of minimally invasive sacroiliac joint fusion: A prospective study. *Med Devices* **6**, 219–229, doi:10.2147/MDER.S55197 (2013).

21. Ledonio, C. G., *et al.* Comparative effectiveness of open versus minimally invasive sacroiliac joint fusion. *Med Devices* **7**, 187–193, doi:10.2147/MDER.S60370 (2014).

22. Shamrock, A. G., *et al.* The safety profile of percutaneous minimally invasive sacroiliac joint fusion. *Global Spine J* **9**, 874–880, doi:10.1177/2192568218816981 (2019).

23. Rudolf, L. Sacroiliac joint arthrodesis MIS technique with titanium implants: Report of the first 50 patients and outcomes. *Open Orthop J* **6**, 495–502, doi:10.2174/1874325001206010495 (2012).

24. Rudolf, L., & Capobianco, R. Five-year clinical and radiographic outcomes after minimally invasive sacroiliac joint fusion using triangular implants. *Open Orthop J* **8**, 375–383, doi:10.2174/1874325001408010375 (2014).

25. Sachs, D., & Capobianco, R. One year successful outcomes for novel sacroiliac joint arthrodesis system. *Ann Surg Innov Res* **6**, 13, doi:10.1186/1750-1164-6-13 (2012).

26. Cummings, J., Jr., & Capobianco, R. A. Minimally invasive sacroiliac joint fusion: One-year outcomes in 18 patients. *Ann Surg Innov Res* **7**, 12, doi:10.1186/1750-1164-7-12 (2013).

27. Duhon, B. S., *et al.* Triangular titanium implants for minimally invasive sacroiliac joint fusion: 2-year follow-up from a prospective multicenter trial. *Int J Spine Surg* **10**, 13, doi:10.14444/3013 (2016).

28. Patel, V., *et al.* Minimally invasive lateral transiliac sacroiliac joint fusion using 3D-printed triangular titanium implants. *Med Devices* **12**, 203–214, doi:10.2147/MDER.S205812 (2019).

29. Khurana, A., *et al.* Percutaneous fusion of the sacroiliac joint with hollow modular anchorage screws: Clinical and radiological outcome. *J Bone Joint Surg Br* **91**, 627–631, doi:10.1302/0301-620X.91B5.21519 (2009).

30. Whang, P. G., *et al.* Long-term prospective clinical and radiographic outcomes after minimally invasive lateral transiliac sacroiliac joint fusion using triangular titanium implants. *Med Devices* **12**, 411–422, doi:10.2147/MDER.S219862 (2019).

31. Heiney, J., *et al.* A systematic review of minimally invasive sacroiliac joint fusion utilizing a lateral transarticular technique. *Int J Spine Surg* **9**, 40, doi:10.14444/2040 (2015).

32. Cross, W. W., *et al.* Minimally invasive sacroiliac joint fusion: 2-year radiographic and clinical outcomes with a principles-based SIJ fusion system. *Open Orthop J* **12**, 7–16, doi:10.2174/1874325001812010007 (2018).

33. Kube, R. A., & Muir, J. M. Sacroiliac joint fusion: One year clinical and radiographic results following minimally invasive sacroiliac joint fusion surgery. *Open Orthop J* **10**, 679–689, doi:10.2174/1874325001610010679 (2016).

34. Martin, C. T., *et al.* Minimally invasive sacroiliac joint fusion: The current evidence. *Int J Spine Surg* **14**, 20–29, doi:10.14444/6072 (2020).

35. Lindsey, D. P., *et al.* Sacroiliac joint fusion minimally affects adjacent lumbar segment motion: A finite element study. *Int J Spine Surg* **9**, 64, doi:10.14444/2064 (2015).

36. Joukar, A., *et al.* Effects on hip stress following sacroiliac joint fixation: A finite element study. *JOR Spine* **2**, e1067, doi:10.1002/jsp2.1067 (2019).

37. Rudolf, L. MIS fusion of the SI joint: Does prior lumbar spinal fusion affect patient outcomes? *Open Orthop J* **7**, 163–168, doi:10.2174/1874325001307010163 (2013).

38. Sachs, D., & Capobianco, R. Minimally invasive sacroiliac joint fusion: One-year outcomes in 40 patients. *Adv Orthop* **2013**, 536128, doi:10.1155/2013/536128 (2013).

39. Gaetani, P., *et al.* Percutaneous arthrodesis of sacro-iliac joint: A pilot study. *J Neurosurg Sci* **57**, 297–301 (2013).

40. Mason, L. W., *et al.* The percutaneous stabilisation of the sacroiliac joint with hollow modular anchorage screws: A prospective outcome study. *Eur Spine J* **22**, 2325–2331, doi:10.1007/s00586-013-2825-2 (2013).

41. Schroeder, J. E., *et al.* Early results of sacro-iliac joint fixation following long fusion to the sacrum in adult spine deformity. *HSS J* **10**, 30–35, doi:10.1007/s11420-013-9374-4 (2014).

42. Sachs, D., *et al.* One-year outcomes after minimally invasive sacroiliac joint fusion with a series of triangular implants: A multicenter, patient-level analysis. *Med Devices* **7**, 299–304, doi:10.2147/MDER.S56491 (2014).

43. Sachs, D., *et al.* Durable intermediate-to long-term outcomes after minimally invasive transiliac sacroiliac joint fusion using triangular titanium implants. *Med Devices* **9**, 213–222, doi:10.2147/MDER.S109276 (2016).

44. Polly, D. W., *et al.* Two-year outcomes from a randomized controlled trial of minimally invasive sacroiliac joint fusion vs. non-surgical management for sacroiliac joint dysfunction. *Int J Spine Surg* **10**, 28, doi:10.14444/3028 (2016).

45. Kancherla, V. K., *et al.* Patient-reported outcomes from sacroiliac joint fusion. *Asian Spine J* **11**, 120–126, doi:10.4184/asj.2017.11.1.120 (2017).

46. Rappoport, L. H., *et al.* Minimally invasive sacroiliac joint fusion using a novel hydroxyapatite-coated screw: Preliminary 1-year clinical and radiographic results of a 2-year prospective study. *World Neurosurg* **101**, 493–497, doi:10.1016/j.wneu.2017.02.046 (2017).

47. Araghi, A., *et al.* Pain and opioid use outcomes following minimally invasive sacroiliac joint fusion with decortication and bone grafting: The Evolusion clinical trial. *Open Orthop J* **11**, 1440–1448, doi:10.2174/1874325001711011440 (2017).

48. Dengler, J. D., *et al.* 1-year results of a randomized controlled trial of conservative management vs. minimally invasive surgical treatment for sacroiliac joint pain. *Pain Physician* **20**, 537–550 (2017).

49. Darr, E., *et al.* Long-term prospective outcomes after minimally invasive trans-iliac sacroiliac joint fusion using triangular titanium implants. *Med Devices* **11**, 113–121, doi:10.2147/MDER.S160989 (2018).

50. Claus, C. F., *et al.* Minimally invasive sacroiliac joint fusion using triangular titanium versus cylindrical threaded implants: A comparison of patient-reported outcomes. *World Neurosurg* **133**, e745–e750, doi:10.1016/j.wneu.2019.09.150 (2020).

20

Posterior fusion

Cory Ullger, Mogana V. Jayakumar, and Navdeep Jassal

Introduction

In recent years, sacroiliac joint (SIJ) dysfunction has become of increasing interest as a source of low back pain. The prevalence of SIJ dysfunction is difficult to assess but is estimated to be as high as 62% in certain populations.[1–3] With increasing awareness of SIJ dysfunction diagnosis in an innovative and dynamic field, minimally invasive surgery (MIS) SIJ fusion systems have become a mainstay treatment option. At the time of writing this text, over 25 SIJ fusion systems that have been approved by the U.S. Food and Drug Administration (FDA) are on the market, and a growing number of them are designed for a posterior approach (Box 20.1).

Open treatment of SIJ dysfunction was described as early as the 1920s, with reports of numerous complications, long recovery times, and poor outcomes, which led to limited adoption of this procedure.[3] Over the last decade, however, significant improvement in implants and surgical techniques has facilitated safer and more effective procedures for the treatment of SIJ dysfunction.[4] In recent years, MIS techniques have gained wide popularity. In 2008, two groups introduced percutaneous approaches to SIJ fusion: Wise and Dall introduced a percutaneous posterior approach[5] and Al-Khayer et al. introduced a percutaneous lateral approach.[6] By 2012, 85% of SIJ fusions were performed using an MIS technique.[7] In 2012, a retrospective case series using dual fiber allograft dowels in an MIS posterior approach demonstrated that nearly 90% of subjects had radiographic stabilization of the joint as well as significant improvement in pain scores.[8] This demonstrated that the posterior allograft technique was possible. Over the past several years it has been refined to be a more minimally invasive approach.

Multiple approaches now exist to fuse the SIJ, the most common being MIS lateral and MIS posterior. Some systems apply a combination of MIS lateral and posterior approaches. Both open posterior and open Smith-Petersen posterolateral transiliac approaches may also still be used in cases where the MIS technique is not an option. This chapter will detail three common posterior approaches to SIJ arthrodesis, two involving stabilization

---

BOX 20.1. FDA-approved MIS SIJ fusion systems for posterior placement

LinQ (PainTEQ)

CornerLoc System (Cornerloc)

Rialto (Medtronic)

PsiF System (Omnia Medical)

SI-DESIS (SI Technology)

Catamaran (SpineSource)

SiJoin (VGI Medical)

TransFasten (Captiva Spine)

SiCure (Alevio Spine)

Sacrix Sacrofuse (KIC Ventures)

DIANA (Signus)

---

with specialized grafts and the other incorporating a cylindrical threaded implant placed via a muscle/tissue-sparing posterior oblique approach using intraoperative stereotactic navigation. Several aspects of the commonly used posterior approaches are compared in Table 20.1.

Posterior SIJ arthrodesis

An MIS posterior approach to SIJ fusion may be performed using fluoroscopic guidance. Image guidance is necessary to plan trajectories and ensure correct placement of instrumentation while minimizing the risk of adjacent nerve and soft tissue damage.

TABLE 20.1 Comparison among commonly used posterior SIJ fusion devices

	LinQ	PsiF System	CornerLoc	Rialto
Allograft	X	X	X	
Large graft window	X			X
No-drill	X			
Single implant	X			
Easy insertion	X	X	X	
Easy-to-use instrumentation	X	X	X	
Clinical data	SECURE study, multi-center and single-center data, biomechanical study, case series	Registry	COVI Study, multi-center, biomechanical study, case series	Case series

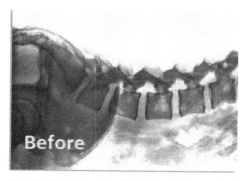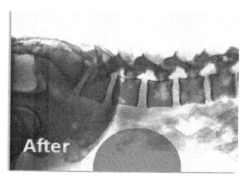

FIGURE 20.1. Leveled-off pelvis with bump placed underneath abdomen. *Source:* Printed with permission from CornerLoc.

This procedure is typically conducted under general anesthesia, although it may be performed under monitored anesthesia care (MAC) anesthesia. The patient is positioned in a prone position (Figure 20.1A) on a radiolucent table (flat-topped or Jackson table) with a large 6- to 8-inch gel bump or blanket roll placed under the umbilicus, lifting the lumbar spine out of lordosis to level off the pelvis and allowing the hips to have 15 to 20 degrees of flexion (Figure 20.1B).

Although the risk of neurologic injury is low with the posterior approach, intraoperative neurophysiology monitoring (IONM) may be performed. Electrodes can be placed on the anterior tibialis, the gastrocnemius, and the rectal sphincter to monitor L5, S1, and S2 nerve roots, respectively.

SIJ fusion performed using fluoroscopic guidance via single graft implant

The patient's skin is sterilized and the patient is draped in the usual fashion, leaving the target hip exposed. center the SIJ being implanted in the center of the fluoroscopy screen. Visually locate the sacrum, ilium, posterior superior iliac spine (PSIS), anterior joint line (AJL), and posterior joint line (PJL). Then, oblique the C-arm contralaterally until the PJL and the AJL are superimposed. This usually occurs between 10 and 35 degrees. The medial and lateral cortical lines of the ilium will start to sharpen as the PJL and AJL start to superimpose.

In the lateral view, make sure the patient is positioned in a true lateral in which a sharp posterior cortical edge is visualized on the sacrum. To see the S1 foramen it may be necessary to tilt the table or wigwag the C-arm to line up the sciatic notches (Figure 20.2A). The S1 foramen is just visible. The guide pin is placed near the S1 foramen. The insertion point for the guide pin needs to be at the midpoint of the joint, just medial to the medial cortical wall of the ilium (Figure 20.2B). Once the insertion point is located, make a simple stab wound there with a scalpel.

The guide pin needs to follow and run parallel to the fluoroscopy beam in order to enter the joint. The target area is the middle third of the joint (Figure 20.3A). This will place the guide pin near the level of the S1 foramen. A correctly placed guide pin is just medial to the medial cortical wall of the ilium.

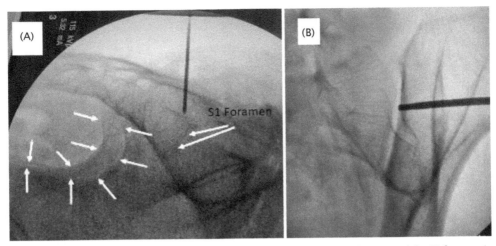

FIGURE 20.2. (**A**) The patient is close to a true lateral as the sciatic notches line up and the S1 foramen is visualized. (**B**) Guide pin insertion at the medial cortical wall of the ilium. *Source:* Printed with permission from PainTEQ.

Preferably, the guide pin will be in a superior to inferior angle in the joint (Figure 20.3B). This will help ensure a perpendicular trajectory into the joint. The perpendicular trajectory is confirmed in the lateral view (Figure 20.3C).

Once the joint space is entered, rotate the C-arm to a lateral to confirm the tip has passed the posterior cortical line (PCL) of the sacrum (Figure 20.4). If it hasn't, then the pin is not in the joint. If the guide pin is past the PCL, it can be gently tapped at this point to advance it further to get good purchase. This will prevent the pin from backing out as the outside and inside dilators are advanced.

The optimal target area for the guide pin is under the PSIS near the S1 foramen (Figure 20.5). The preferred angle is closest to the line that is perpendicular to the posterior sacral line (Figure 20.6). If the angle is too shallow, the upper tongs won't engage into the joint.

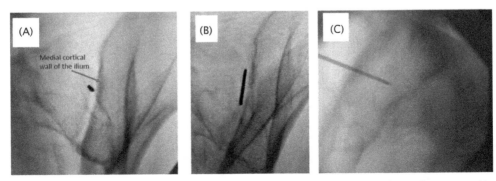

FIGURE 20.3. (**A**) The target area demonstrated in the middle of the joint. (**B**) Guide pin demonstrated in a superior to inferior angle. (**C**) Confirmation of the perpendicular trajectory in lateral view. *Source:* Printed with permission from PainTEQ.

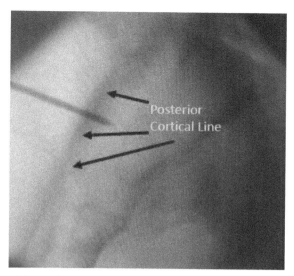

FIGURE 20.4. The tip of the guide pin has passed the posterior cortical line of the sacrum. *Source:* Printed with permission from PainTEQ.

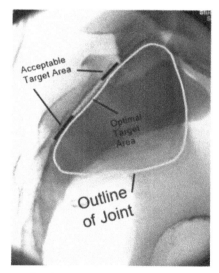

FIGURE 20.5. Optimal target area for the guide pin. *Source:* Printed with permission from PainTEQ.

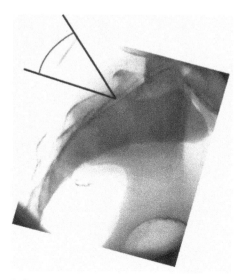

FIGURE 20.6. Preferred angle for the guide pin. *Source:* Printed with permission from PainTEQ.

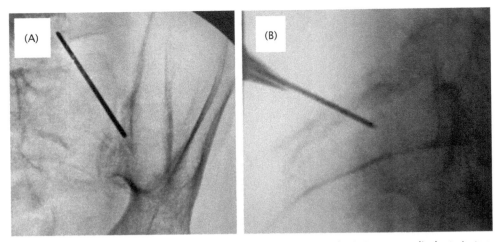

FIGURE 20.7. (**A**) Guide pin in a superior to inferior orientation. (**B**) Guide pin in a perpendicular trajectory on lateral view. *Source:* Printed with permission from PainTEQ.

Direct the guide pin in a superior to inferior orientation (Figure 20.7A). This angulation will bring the guide pin closer to a perpendicular trajectory to the sacrum on the lateral view (Figure 20.7B).

Once correct GP placement has been confirmed on the lateral, the incision can be made (Figure 20.8A). The incision needs to be long enough to accommodate the width of the outside dilator. The surgeon can draw a line from tong to tong on the outside dilator to mark the incision (Figure 20.8B).

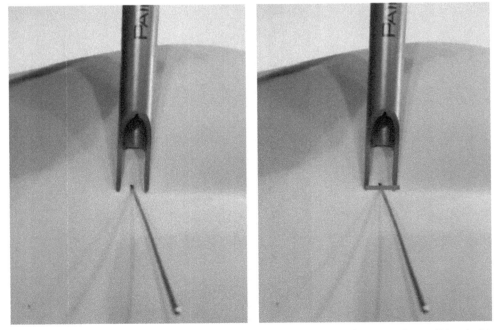

FIGURE 20.8. (**A**) Incision preparation. (**B**) Marking the incision between the tongs. *Source:* Printed with permission from PainTEQ.

The next step involves making the incision and channel. The tendons and ligaments need to be cleared. This can be done by running the #10 blade scalpel along the caudal and cephalic sides of the guide pin all the way to the joint (Figure 20.9). Clearing the ligaments is important because they can hold up the dilators.

After the channel is made, the next step involves placement of the dilators. The inside and outside dilators should be handed to the surgeon separately to prevent the outside one from being dropped (Figure 20.10). The surgeon will slide the inside dilator into the outside one. The instruments are keyholed. The inside dilator has a guide rail that will slide down the alignment slot in the outer dilator. This ensures that the instruments can only be correctly paired up.

Advance the dilators down the guide pin by gently tapping them with a mallet. Use lateral fluoroscopic imaging to track the depth of the dilators (Figure 20.11). Stop the advance once the dilator tongs reach the PCL of the sacrum. Bring the C-arm back around to the original oblique angle.

Angle the C-arm cephalically a few degrees so the upper tong can be viewed. The tong should lie just medial to the medial cortical wall of the ilium (Figure 20.12). If the tong isn't just medial to the ilium, turn the dilators so that it is positioned correctly.

Next, tilt the C-arm caudally until the bottom tong can be visualized (Figure 20.13). Ensure the bottom tong is aligned with the posterior joint line. If it isn't, turn the dilators so that it is positioned correctly. Once the tong is lined up with the posterior joint, rotate the C-arm back to lateral.

Advance the dilators by gently tapping on them with a mallet until the hard stop on the outside dilator meets the PCL of the sacrum (Figure 20.14). Once the dilators are fully

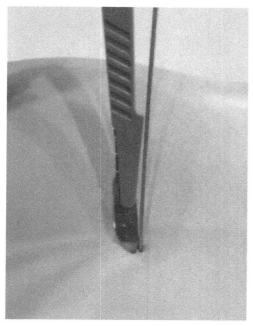
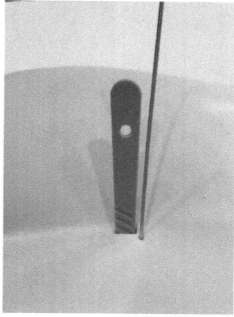

FIGURE 20.9. Scalpel along the caudal and cephalic sides of the guide pin all the way down to the joint.
Source: Printed with permission from PainTEQ.

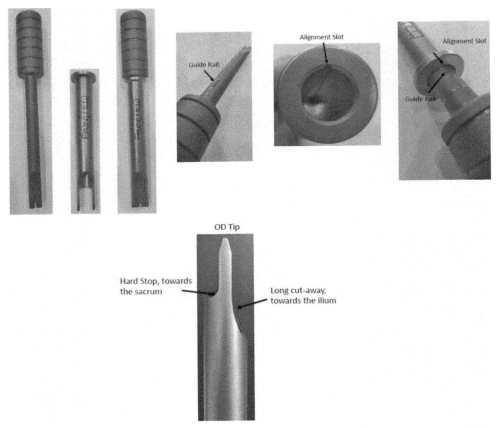

FIGURE 20.10. Inside dilator and outside dilator orientation. *Source:* Printed with permission from PainTEQ.

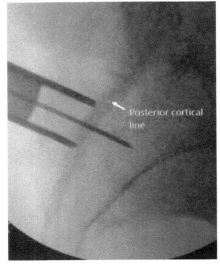

FIGURE 20.11. Depth of the dilators in the lateral view. Advancement is stopped once the dilator tongs reach the posterior cortical line of the sacrum. *Source:* Printed with permission from PainTEQ.

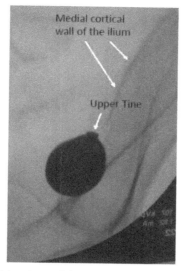

FIGURE 20.12. Upper tong medial to the medial cortical wall of the ilium. *Source:* Printed with permission from PainTEQ.

seated on the sacrum, remove the inside dilator. At this point the outside dilator becomes a working channel.

Rotate the C-arm around to an AP. Next, we want to get a "barrel shot" to confirm the working channel is in the joint. The first shot in the AP usually shows the working channel in an oblique orientation from a superior to inferior trajectory (Figure 20.15A). Tilt the C-arm cephalically until the working channel orients into a 9 o'clock and 3 o'clock orientation

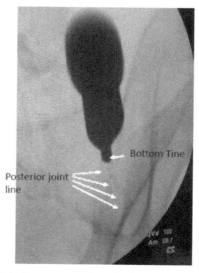

FIGURE 20.13. Visualization of the bottom tong aligned with the posterior joint line. *Source:* Printed with permission from PainTEQ.

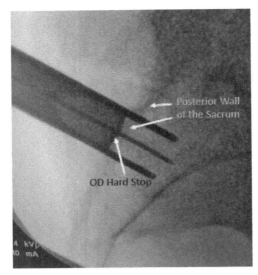

FIGURE 20.14. Outside dilator hard stop meeting the posterior cortical line of the sacrum. *Source:* Printed with permission from PainTEQ.

(Figure 20.15B). The x-ray technician needs to keep the working channel centered in the fluoroscopic screen.

Once the working channel is orientated in a 9 o'clock/3 o'clock trajectory, rotate the C-arm over so the fluoroscopic beam shoots straight down the working channel tube (Figure 20.16). In this view the joint should be visualized in the middle of the channel. If it can't be viewed, you may not be in the joint and may need to start over. Based on patient anatomy, it seldom occurs that the joint can't be viewed through the working channel, but the channel is in the joint. If the joint can't be viewed, check the channel's orientation. If the orientation

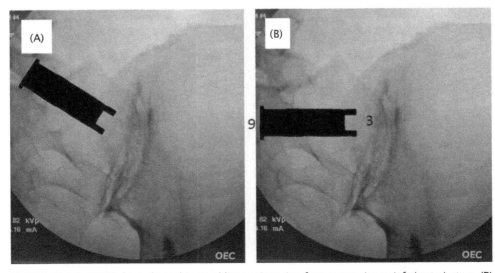

FIGURE 20.15. (A) Working channel in an oblique orientation from a superior to inferior trajectory. **(B)** Working channel in 9 o'clock/3 o'clock orientation. *Source:* Printed with permission from PainTEQ.

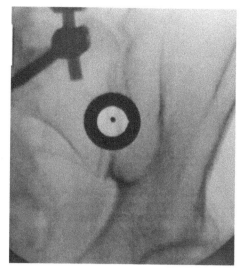

FIGURE 20.16. Fluoroscopic beam co-axial down the working channel tube. *Source:* Printed with permission from PainTEQ.

and trajectory look correct in the oblique view and the joint was entered with minimal malleting, then continue on to the next step and rotate the C-arm into a lateral.

Place the joint decorticator into the working channel, ensuring that the guide rail and the alignment slot are lined up. Advance the decorticator by tapping it forward with a mallet until the handle meets the working channel or the decorticator tip arrives at the anterior cortical line of the sacrum (Figure 20.17). This decorticates the joint and creates an implant bed.

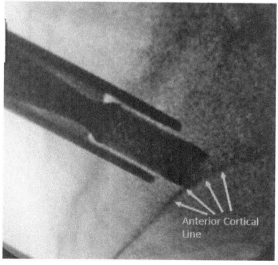

FIGURE 20.17. Tip of the joint decorticator at the anterior cortical line of the sacrum. *Source:* Printed with permission from PainTEQ.

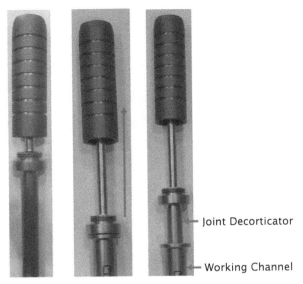

Joint Decorticator

Working Channel

FIGURE 20.18. Unscrewing the joint decorticator by turning the handle. *Source:* Printed with permission from PainTEQ.

To remove the joint decorticator, turn the handle counterclockwise to unscrew it (Figure 20.18). The handle is now a slap hammer. Start the handle with it all the way down and quickly and forcefully extend it along the shaft. Repeat the last step until the decorticator has come out of the working channel.

Then, place the cortical bone implant into the inserter (Figure 20.19). The tongs on the inserter will slide into the groves on the implant. Fully seat the implant into the tongs. Once

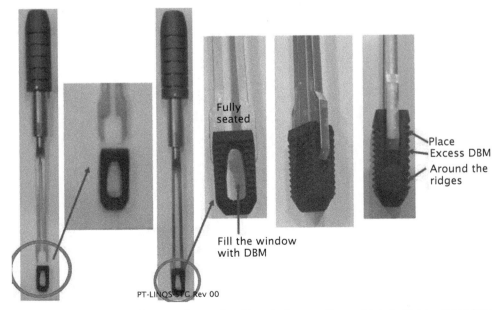

Fully seated

Place
Excess DBM
Around the ridges

Fill the window with DBM

PT-LINQS-STG Rev 00

FIGURE 20.19. The cortical bone implant is placed into the inserter. *Source:* Printed with permission from PainTEQ.

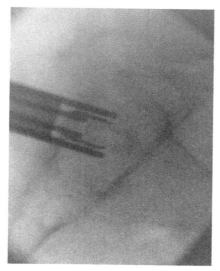

FIGURE 20.20. Implant fully seated into the implant bed. *Source:* Printed with permission from PainTEQ.

the implant is fully seated, fill the window with the demineralized bone matrix (DBM). Loosely place the excess DBM around the implant ridges.

To insert the cortical implant, slide the loaded inserter into the working channel, ensuring the rail guide and the alignment slot are lined up. Advance the inserter by gently tapping with a mallet until it is fully seated into the implant bed (Figure 20.20). Once the implant is fully seated, remove the inserter and working channel.

The implant is properly placed if it lies in between the ilium and sacrum in the posterior aspect of the SIJ (Figure 20.21).

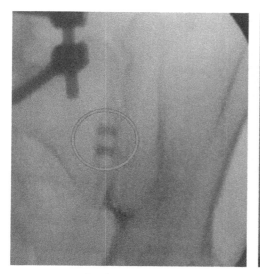
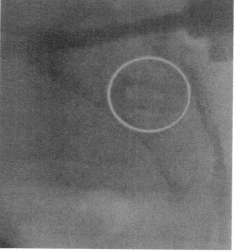

FIGURE 20.21. Final images depicting the properly placed implant. *Source:* Printed with permission from PainTEQ.

SIJ fusion performed using fluoroscopic guidance via dual graft implants

The patient's skin is sterilized and the patient is draped in the usual fashion, leaving the target hip exposed. A C-arm image scanner intensifier is used to obtain a true AP view of the SIJ. The C-arm is rotated to a medial to lateral oblique orientation of 15 to 20 degrees from the AP plane over the operative SIJ until the joint line becomes clearly visible.

Using a Steinmann pin as an opaque fluoroscopic marker, locate a line from cephalad to caudal in the orientation of the joint line, and mark the skin along that line (Figure 20.22A). Next, locate the cephalad and caudal apex of the SIJ, marking a 3-cm line medial to lateral over each apex (Figure 20.22B). Then, mark a 2-cm entry line 1 cm medial and 1 cm cephalad to the superior site, and mark another site 0.5 to 1 cm medial and 1 cm caudal to the inferior site (Figure 20.22C).

To optimize SIJ immobilization and stability, use two grafts. Place the pin for the upper graft into the SIJ just lateral to the L5–S1 facet joint, within and down the trajectory of the SIJ. Place the lower pin directly caudal to the protuberance of the PSIS, within and up into the trajectory of the SIJ (Figure 20.23A). Use a small mallet to advance the pins into the joint space 1.5 to 2 cm, and move the C-arm to a lateral position for confirmation. The two pins should be in intersecting planes at 70 to 90 degrees to each other in the AP plane as seen from a lateral view (Figure 20.23B). If adjustments need to be made, move the C-arm back to an oblique AP view to make adjustments, once again moving to a lateral view to confirm the desired placement.

Once ready to move to the instrumentation steps, leave the C-arm in the lateral position for confirmation during the instrumentation steps.

Regarding site preparation, once the graft sites have been selected and the 2.4-mm × 9-inch Steinmann pins have been placed, proceed with placing the T-handle onto the finder by pulling back on the quick-connect collet and releasing it once the T-handle is seated and the arms of the T-handle are aligned with the feet of the finder (Figure 20.24A). Then, place the finder over either the superior or inferior Steinmann pin, ensuring that the top of the pin is placed into the very tip of the finder (Figure 20.24B). The pin cannot be swept into the groove from the side. Ensure the longer cutaway inclined side of the finder tip faces the

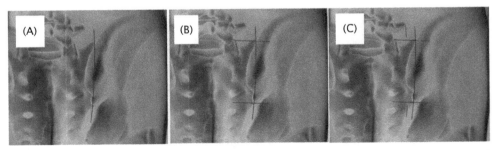

FIGURE 20.22. (A) Pin in cephalad to caudal line in the orientation of the joint line. (B) Cephalad and caudal apex of the SIJ is located, marking a 3-cm line medial to lateral over each apex. (C) 2-cm entry line 1 cm medial and 1 cm cephalad to the superior site is marked, and another site is marked 0.5 to 1 cm medial and 1 cm caudal to the inferior site. *Source:* Printed with permission from CornerLoc.

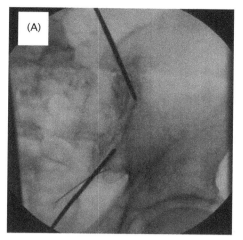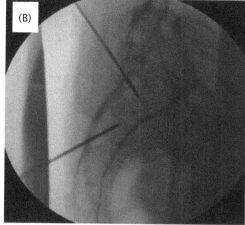

FIGURE 20.23. (A) Advancing the two pins into the joint space. (B) Lateral view with pins confirmed in the joint space. *Source:* Printed with permission from CornerLoc.

ilium. Advance until the shorter stop shelf side of the finder tip bottoms out on the sacrum (Figure 20.24C).

Next, place the retraction guide tube over the finder and engage it into the joint space with the longer incline side toward the ilium and the shorter stop shelf tip of the finder toward the sacrum. First, use the lines on the side of the finder to orient the feet of the retraction guide tube in line with the joint space (Figure 20.25A). Slide the retraction guide tube down the finder into the soft tissue until the feet reach the SIJ. The hammer tube is then used to impact the retraction guide tube into the joint space (Figure 20.25B). Gently impact the retraction guide tube until its shorter stop shelf contacts the sacrum (Figure 20.25C). Remove the finder and the Steinmann pin.

The next step involves using the drill. The CornerLoc drill cuts both on the tip and the sides as it emerges from the end of the retraction guide tube and into the SIJ space (Figure 20.26A). Ensure the drill is rotating in a forward direction. Allowing the drill to do

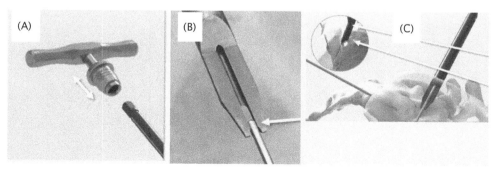

FIGURE 20.24. (A) Placement of the T-handle onto the finder. (B) Placement of the finder over the Steinmann pin. (C) Advance until the shorter stop shelf side of the finder tip bottoms out on the sacrum. *Source:* Printed with permission from CornerLoc.

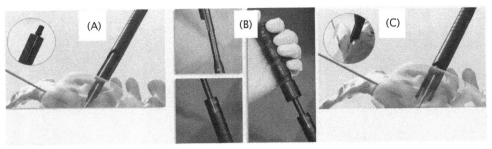

FIGURE 20.25. (**A**) Slide the retraction guide tube down the finder until the feet reach the SIJ. (**B**) Use the hammer tube to impact the retraction guide tube into the joint space. (**C**) Impact the retraction guide tube until its shorter stop shelf contacts the sacrum. *Source:* Printed with permission from CornerLoc.

the work, slowly drill down into the joint space until the drill stop contacts the top of the retraction guide tube (Figure 20.26B). Keep the drill in forward rotation, and withdraw the drill from the joint and out of the guide tube, releasing the power trigger as the drill flutes emerge from the top of the guide tube. The drill creates a rounded channel along the medial side of the PSIS and into the joint (Figure 20.26C).

The next step involves the square broach. To properly orient the broach cutting feature, insert the square broach into the retraction guide tube, aligning the key bump located on the side of the broach shaft with the keyed slot on the inside of the retraction guide tube (Figure 20.27A). Advance the broach until the handle stop contacts the top of the retraction guide tube (Figure 20. 27B). In patients with lower bone density, surgeons may elect to broach to a lesser depth at their discretion. Once broaching is complete, remove the broach using the slap hammer to ensure integrity of the square hole shape (Figure 20.27C). The graft site is now square and ready to receive the CornerLoc DBM sponge and CornerLoc cortical graft (Figure 20.27D).

The next step involves graft placement. Place the CornerLoc DBM sponge (9 mm^3) in the inserter by gently squeezing it and pressing it into the end of the inserter, and insert it into the retraction guide tube (Figure 20.28A). Once the inserter stop contacts the top of the tube, push the DBM sponge into the graft hole with the final impactor. Place the CornerLoc cortical graft (8 mm × 8 mm × 20.6 mm) into the end of the inserter by placing the graft in

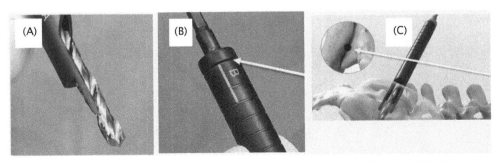

FIGURE 20.26. (**A**) Drill. (**B**) Drill emerging from end of retraction guide tube. placement of the finder over the Steinmann (**C**) The drill creates a rounded channel along the medial side of the PSIS and into the joint. *Source:* Printed with permission from CornerLoc.

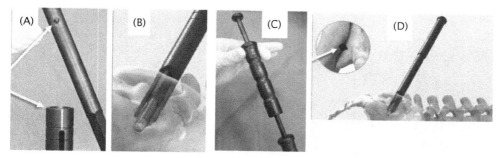

FIGURE 20.27. (**A**) Insert the square broach into the retraction guide tube, aligning the key bump located on the side of the broach shaft with the keyed slot on the inside of the retraction guide tube. (**B**) Advance the broach until the handle stop contacts the top of the retraction guide tube. (**C, D**) Remove the broach using the slap hammer to ensure integrity of the square hole shape. *Source:* Printed with permission from CornerLoc.

the graft holder on the sterile surgical back table, while pressing the inserter down over the graft until it snaps into place (Figure 20.28B,C).

Place the inserter down the retraction guide tube, keeping the key bump and key slot aligned (Figure 20.28D). Tap gently with a mallet to seat the graft. Once the inserter stop

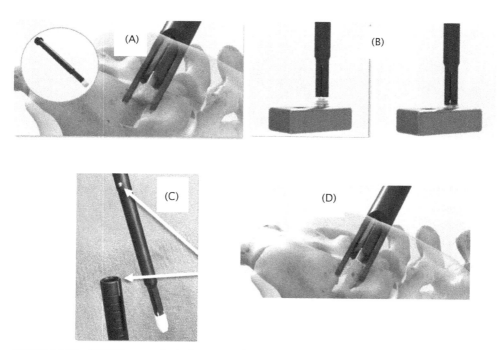

FIGURE 20.28. (**A**) DBM sponge in the inserter and is positioned it into the retraction guide tube. Once the inserter stop contacts the top of the tube, the DBM sponge is pushed into the graft hole with the final impactor. (**B, C**) Cortical graft is placed into the end of the inserter. (**C**) Inserter is placed down the retraction guide tube, keeping the key bump and key slot aligned. (**D**) Graft is seated by tapping gently with mallet. Once the inserter stop contacts the top of the tube, the cortical graft is tapped into the graft hole using the final impactor and a small mallet. *Source:* Printed with permission from CornerLoc.

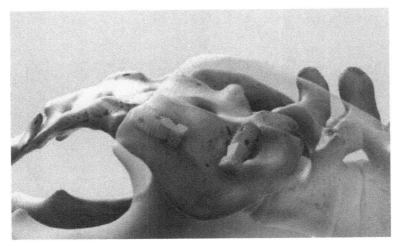

FIGURE 20.29. Graft in place. *Source:* Printed with permission from CornerLoc.

contacts the top of the tube, tap the CornerLoc cortical graft into the graft hole using the final impactor and a small mallet (Figure 20.28).

Once the graft is satisfactorily in place, remove the inserter, final impactor, and re-traction guide tube. Hemostasis is applied and the wound is closed per surgeon preference. Figure 20.29 shows the graft in place.

SIJ fusion performed using fluoroscopic guidance via cylindrical threaded implant and intraoperative stereotactic navigation

This section will describe the surgical technique for this procedure.[9]

A small incision is made over the contralateral PSIS, and a percutaneous reference frame is placed for the StealthStation navigation system (Medtronic). After confirmation, a three-dimensional O-arm spin is performed, with the information subsequently trans-ferred to the StealthStation for navigation. The ipsilateral SIJ is localized with navigation and decorticated with a large tap to facilitate the placement of allograft for direct arthrod-esis. The navigation is used to localize entry points and trajectories for the placement of two cylindrical threaded implants (CTIs) across the SIJ. Two small incisions are made at predetermined locations, and following navigated pilot holes, two allograph-filled CTIs are implanted with the assistance of navigation. Optimal placement of the CTIs is across the SIJ while avoiding any breach in the sacral foramina. Final placement is confirmed with an additional three-dimensional O-arm spin.

The device can be implanted under either navigation or fluoroscopy. The following illustrates fluoroscopic imaging for this approach. The patient is positioned prone on a Jackson table. The C-arm is angled 30 degrees cephalic from standard AP. The angle will vary by patient but should be perpendicular to the sacral inclination. An acceptable radiograph will identify the S1 foramen. This view can be used to determine the initial starting point cephalic to caudal (Figure 20.30A). An acceptable radiograph will demonstrate posterior

(A)

(B)

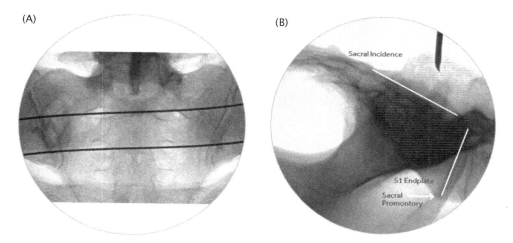

FIGURE 20.30. (**A**) S1 foramina. (**B**) Orientation of the S1 endplate, the approximate sacral incidence, and the sacral promontory. *Source:* Printed with permission from Medtronic.

and anterior walls of the sacrum. This view can be used to determine the orientation of the S1 endplate, the approximate sacral incidence, and the sacral promontory. The trajectory in this plane should be directed at, or inferior to, the sacral promontory (Figure 20.30B).

The oblique views are taken with the C-arm positioned at a 25- to 30-degree angle to the AP plane. An acceptable radiograph will demonstrate a closely collimated, centered SI joint with the anterior and posterior joint margins superimposed. The left posterior oblique view demonstrates the right SIJ as the side up, and the right posterior oblique view demonstrates the left SIJ side up. This view can show the lateral aspect of the PSIS. This will be the site of the incision (Figure 20.31).

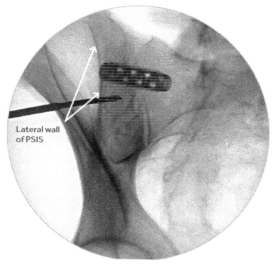

FIGURE 20.31. Site of incision. *Source:* Printed with permission from Medtronic.

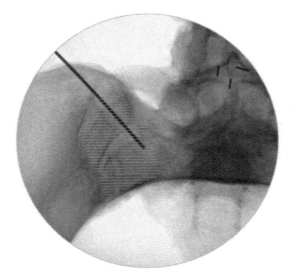

FIGURE 20.32. The sacral inlet view. *Source:* Printed with permission from Medtronic.

The sacral inlet view is taken with the C-arm typically positioned at a 25- to 30-degree angle caudally to the AP plane (Figure 20.32). An acceptable radiograph will demonstrate the complete, circular pelvic ring. Anatomically, this plane will be parallel to the anterior sacrum, and thus the actual angle of the C-arm may vary. This view is critical in confirming depth and avoiding violation of the anterior pelvic rim.

Confirmation of final placement should be examined in three views: lateral, sacral inlet, and sacral outlet (Figure 20.33). If it is determined the guide wire has advanced, stop and verify instrumentation in all three views.

Safety and complications

MIS posterior SIJ fusion has been shown to have an improved safety profile compared to open and MIS lateral approaches. Open fusion complications include increased rates of blood loss during surgery, pseudoarthrosis, deep wound infection, and painful hardware. In a multi-center study that compared open versus MIS SIJ fusion, estimated blood loss, operating time, and length of hospitalization were significantly lower for MIS fusion as compared to open approaches.[10] Ledonio et al. also demonstrated similar results in a retrospective single-site study when examining the safety and efficacy of MIS SIJ fusion compared to open approaches.[11]

With a lateral MIS approach there is the risk of injuring the gluteal musculature or impinging the sacral nerve roots as they exit their neural foramen, as well as roots within the canal itself. Care must be taken to stay lateral to the neural foramen to avoid this and to employ imaging and IONM when placing hardware. Some retrospective case studies have shown that no serious adverse events have occurred, including orthopedic, neurologic, and vascular complications.[12,13] A posterior approach is less invasive as it allows for

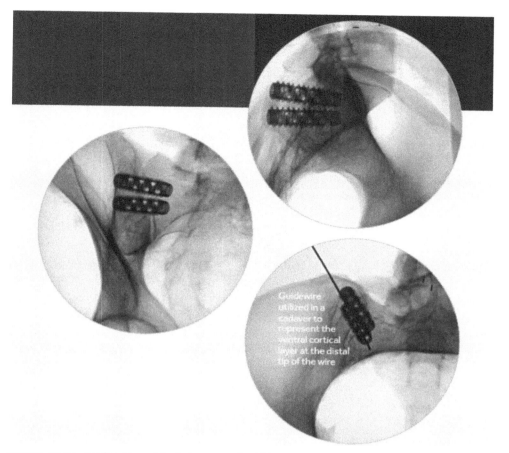

FIGURE 20.33. Confirmation of final placement should be examined in three views: lateral, sacral inlet, and sacral outlet. *Source:* Printed with permission from Medtronic.

simple access to the SIJ, which eliminates transgluteal risks in addition to the risks of a hematoma or nerve injury. There is also a significant improvement in surgical time compared to other approaches. This approach is associated with reduced morbidity, as patients do not have weight-bearing restrictions and recover more quickly. The posterior approach allows for simple access to the SIJ, which expedites surgical time and recovery.

Efficacy and evidence

The majority of the literature, including several randomized controlled trials, provides extensive data supporting the efficacy of the lateral MIS approach as discussed in Chapter 19.

Martin et al. in 2020 published an extensive review of the current literature for lateral and posterior MIS SIJ fusion.[14] In it they provide a pooled analysis of all existing data, showing a mean decrease of 80.3 to 32.2 on a 100-point visual analog scale (VAS) and a mean decrease of 56.2 to 34.4 on the Oswestry Disability Index (ODI). They conclude that

MIS SIJ fusion provides significant improvement in pain scores and disability in most patients. Of note, this study pooled data from the lateral and posterior surgical approaches but did not compare one to the other.

As MIS approaches to SIJ fusion continue to develop, they have evolved from being a viable alternative to open surgical approaches to becoming routine practice and standard of care. As evidenced in a 2014 study by Lorio et al. that surveyed 121 surgeons from the International Society for the Advancement of Spine Surgery (ISASS) and Society for Minimally Invasive Spine Surgery (SMISS), from 2009 to 2012, the percentage of MIS procedures increased from 39% to 87%.[15] This study demonstrated several advantages of MIS techniques over open techniques, including a reported decrease in length of stay from 4.33 days for open surgical procedures to 1.69 days for MIS procedures, as well as decreased operating room times and clinical improvement in pain scores.

Advantages of minimally invasive SIJ fusion over open surgical technique have been demonstrated in further studies as well. In a 2013 multi-center, retrospective comparative cohort study by Smith et al., the operative time averaged 163 ± 25 minutes for open surgical fusion versus 70 ± 24 minutes for MIS SIJ fusion.[10] At 2-year follow-up, 47% of the patients in the open fusion group and 82% of the patients in the MIS group had substantial clinical benefit as evidenced by pain scores. The success of MIS strategies over open SIJ fusion was again replicated in a 2019 analysis of two Level 1 randomized controlled trials in which Yson et al. showed that MIS approaches have lower morbidity and shorter recovery time.[16]

In a 2014 retrospective analysis, Ledonio et al. showed that MIS SIJ fusion techniques were associated with significantly lower estimated blood loss (41 ± 31 mL) than open joint fusion (681 ± 479 mL).[17] This study showed significant improvement in ODI scores for both the MIS and open fusion groups, with no significant difference in mean postoperative scores between the groups. However, one of the limitations noted in this study was that ODI scores may be confounded by concomitant spine issues. Another limitation noted was the lack of postoperative radiographic evidence of successful SIJ fusion, which is postulated to be lower in MIS approaches as compared to open surgical approaches.

A prospective multi-center cohort study in Germany published by Fuchs in 2018 compared computed tomography (CT) scans from before surgery, after surgery, and more than 6 months of follow-up from 115 operations and found that only 31.3% were assessed by the radiologist as unequivocally fused.[18] The authors hypothesize that bony fusion may not have completed by the 6-month follow-up, as evidenced by bone progression in patients who had later CT scans. In addition, this paper showed no significant correlation between fusion rates and clinical findings, indicating that acceptable SIJ stability can be achieved even with delayed fusion.

There are a number of reports based on the Sacroiliac Joint Fusion with iFuse Implant System (SIFI) trial, a prospective, multi-center single-arm clinical trial that analyzed cases using the iFuse Implant System, a series of triangular titanium implants. In a 2016 report by Duhon et al., 172 patients were enrolled and treated with the minimally invasive iFuse Implant System; 138 of them met criteria for a composite of successful treatment. There was a statistically significant reduction in pain scores at every follow-up time point from 6 months to 24 months.[19]

As part of the 2014 INSITE (investigation of Sacroiliac Fusion Treatment) trial, Whang et al. conducted a prospective randomized controlled trial comparing SIJ fusion using triangular implants to nonsurgical management of SIJ pain and found superior 6-month outcomes in patients who underwent SIJ fusion.[20] Nonsurgical management in this study included pain medications, physical therapy, SIJ steroid injections, and radiofrequency ablation of sacral nerve roots, while SIJ fusion was done using an MIS lateral transiliac approach with the iFuse Implant System using fluoroscopy or three-dimensional computer navigation based on intraoperative CT imaging. At the 6-month post-intervention follow-up, 81.5% of SIJ fusion patients met the study's primary success end point, as compared to only 23.9% of patients from the nonsurgical management group. Crossover from the nonsurgical management group was permitted after the initial 6-month end point for patients who did not experience adequate pain relief.

Another publication based on the same randomized controlled trial dataset from the INSITE trial was published in 2016 by Polly et al. and showed that 82% of patients assigned to the SIJ fusion group met threshold improvements from baseline in SIJ pain by the VAS and ODI scores, while less than 10% of subjects in the nonsurgical management group met substantial improvement thresholds.[21]

A long-term follow-up study by Darr et al. in 2018 reported clinical, functional, and safety outcomes from participants in the SIFI and INSITE prospective clinical trials at a 3-year postoperative follow-up period.[22] In this study, 86% of patients who underwent MIS SIJ fusion procedures met the primary efficacy success end point, and there were significant improvements in SIJ pain score as well as ODI at the 3-year follow-up. Patients reported satisfaction with the iFuse MIS result in 96% of treated cases, which correlated with improvements in SIJ pain score and ODI.

As previously mentioned, most available datasets prove success with the lateral approach to SIJ fusion and indicate that further investigation is required to see if the results are reproducible with the posterior approach. At the current time, there is minimal evidence in the literature supporting the direct posterior approach with graft implantation. There are two ongoing randomized controlled trials involving biomechanical studies using the posterior approach. Early data from these biomechanical studies show significantly decreased motion in the joint associated with immediate fixation. Future directions in research are promising. The SECURE study (Single Arm, Multicenter, Prospective, Clinical Study on a Novel Minimally Invasive Posterior Sacroiliac Fusion Device) is currently enrolling patients. This is a prospective 12-month study of 150 patients involving scientific investigators across the United States. The purpose is to investigate the safety and efficacy using the PainTeq LinQ device.

The CornerLoc system is one of the FDA-approved MIS SIJ fusion systems for posterior placement. A novel clinical trial is recruiting participants with refractory SIJ dysfunction in order to compare the safety and efficacy of the CornerLoc SI Joint Stabilization System to intraarticular SIJ injection, the current standard of care.[23] This study is a randomized, open-label crossover trial that is enrolling patients across multiple centers. Patients will first be randomized to either receive the CornerLoc SI Joint Stabilization Procedure or an SIJ steroid injection. Six months after the initial procedure, the efficacy rate (measured as the percentage of patients who report ≥50% improvement in pain) will be determined as the primary outcome measure. Secondary outcome measures include quality-of-life improvement (based on the Patient-Reported Outcomes Measurement Information System [PROMIS-29] survey) and several measures of clinical improvement (including those measured by the ODI, the Timed Up and Go test, the Zurich Claudication Questionnaire, and medication use). Patients who fail to respond to the initial randomized treatment assignment at 6 months will receive the nonrandomized treatment in the crossover phase of the trial.

The SECURE trial is a prospective, multisite, prospective, single-arm study that examines the outcomes associated with the treatment of sacroiliac disease with the LinQ fusion procedure. Data collected will include VAS. Self-report questionnaires will be administered, including the ODI to measure low back pain and disability and the PROMIS 29 survey to measure physical, mental, and social health and well-being.

References

1. Schwarzer AC, et al. The sacroiliac joint in chronic low back pain. *Spine.* 1995;20(1):31–37.
2. Sembrano JN, Polly DW. How often is low back pain not coming from the back. *Spine.* 2009;34(1):E27–E32.
3. Tran ZV, et al. Sacroiliac joint fusion methodology—minimally invasive compared to screw-type surgeries: A systematic review and meta-analysis. *Pain Physician.* 2019;22:29–40.
4. Rajpal S, Burneikiene S. Minimally invasive sacroiliac joint fusion with cylindrical threaded implants using intraoperative stereotactic navigation. *World Neurosurg.* 2019;122:e1588–e1591.
5. International Society for the Advancement of Spinal Surgery. Statement on coding changes for minimally invasive SI joint fusion. http://www.isass.org/public_policy/2013-08-07-isass-statement-minimally-invasive-si-joint-fusion-coding-changes.html
6. Al-Khayer A, et al. Percutaneous sacroiliac joint arthrodesis: A novel technique. *J Spinal Disord Tech.* 2008;21:359–363. doi:10.1097/BSD.0b013e318145ab96
7. Cleveland AW, et al. Mini-open sacroiliac joint fusion with direct bone grafting and minimally invasive fixation using intraoperative navigation. *J Spine Surg.* 2019;5:31–37. doi:10.21037/jss.2019.01.04
8. McGuire RA, et al. Dual fibular allograft dowel technique for sacroiliac joint arthrodesis. *Evid Based Spine Care J.* 2012;3(3):21–28. doi:10.1055/s-0032-1327806
9. Claus CF, et al. Minimally invasive sacroiliac joint fusion using triangular titanium versus cylindrical threaded implants: A comparison of patient-reported outcomes. *World Neurosurg.* 2020;133:e745–e750. doi:10.1016/j.wneu.2019.09.150. PMID: 31605853.
10. Smith AG, et al. Open versus minimally invasive sacroiliac joint fusion: A multi-center comparison of perioperative measures and clinical outcomes. *Annals Surg Innov Res.* 2013;7(1):14. https://doi.org/10.1186/1750-1164-7-14
11. Ledonio CG, et al. Minimally invasive versus open sacroiliac joint fusion: Are they similarly safe and effective? *Clin Orthop Relat Res.* 2014;472(6):1831–1838.
12. Willits M, et al. Safety and efficacy of posterior approach SI stabilization and fusion with specialized grafts. North American Neuromodulation Society annual meeting, September 2018.
13. Dhuram M, et al. Pain reduction at 12 months after posterior approach SI stabilization and fusion with specialized graft: 10 case series. American Society for Pain and Neuroscience annual meeting, July 2019.
14. Martin CT, et al. Minimally invasive sacroiliac joint fusion: The current evidence. *Int J Spine Surg.* 2020;14:20–29. doi:10.14444/6072

15. Lorio MP, et al. Utilization of minimally invasive surgical approach for sacroiliac joint fusion in surgeon population of ISASS and SMISS membership. *Open Orthop J.* 2014;8:1–6. https://doi.org/10.2174/1874325001408010001

16. Yson SC, et al. Sacroiliac joint fusion: Approaches and recent outcomes. *PM&R.* 2019;S1:S114–S117. doi:10.1002/pmrj.12198

17. Ledonio CG, et al. Minimally invasive versus open sacroiliac joint fusion: Are they similarly safe and effective? *Clin Orthop Rel Res.* 2014;472(6):1831–1838. https://doi.org/10.1007/s11999-014-3499-8

18. Fuchs V, Ruhl B. Distraction arthrodesis of the sacroiliac joint: 2-year results of a descriptive prospective multi-center cohort study in 171 patients. *Eur Spine J.* 2018;27:194–204. https://doi.org/10.1007/s00586-017-5313-2

19. Duhon BS, et al. Triangular titanium implants for minimally invasive sacroiliac joint fusion: 2-year follow-up from a prospective multicenter trial. *Int J Spine Surg.* 2016;10:13. https://doi.org/10.14444/3013

20. Whang P, et al. Sacroiliac joint fusion using triangular titanium implants vs. non-surgical management: Six-month outcomes from a prospective randomized controlled trial. *Int J Spine Surg.* 2015;9:6. https://doi.org/10.14444/2006

21. Polly DW, et al. Two-year outcomes from a randomized controlled trial of minimally invasive sacroiliac joint fusion vs. non-surgical management for sacroiliac joint dysfunction. *Int J Spine Surg.* 2016;10:28. https://doi.org/10.14444/3028

22. Darr E, et al. Long-term prospective outcomes after minimally invasive trans-iliac sacroiliac joint fusion using triangular titanium implants. *Med Devices.* 2018;11:113–121. https://doi.org/10.2147/MDER.S160989

23. Fishman M. Comparison of CornerLoc SI Joint Stabilization and steroid injections for sacroiliac joint dysfunction. https://clinicaltrials.gov/ct2/show/study/NCT04218838

21

Postoperative care

Usman Latif, Tyler Concannon, and Andrew Frazier

Introduction

Sacroiliac joint (SIJ) fusion can be undertaken via an open surgical technique or a minimally invasive surgical (MIS) technique. The open surgical technique may consist of an anterior or posterior approach followed by bone harvesting and grafting along with a plate, typically secured with three screws. The MIS technique can be a lateral or posterior approach. The lateral approach is typically performed with the placement of three triangular plasma-sprayed ingrowth fusion rods (iFuse Implant System; SI-BONE, Inc, San Jose, CA, USA). The posterior MIS approach can be performed with the use of hardware, such as cages or screws, or using percutaneously placed small bone allograft into the SIJ (LinQ SI Joint Stabilization System; PainTEQ, Tampa, FL, USA).

One of the most noticeable benefits, aside from improved pain and disability outcomes, when comparing MIS SIJ fusion to the open surgical technique, is the dramatically reduced recovery time. The combination of reduced operative time with decreased blood loss and hospital length of stay has led to decreased complication rates and improvement in patient recovery. In this chapter, we will discuss postoperative recommendations, including ambulation, wound care, antibiotic guidelines, and follow-up interval, for patients who have undergone open surgical SIJ fusion versus MIS SIJ fusion.

Ambulation guidelines

Following any surgical procedure, early ambulation is always a physician-directed goal to help prevent complications such as deep venous thrombosis and pulmonary embolism. Following open SIJ fusion, it is recommended that patients are toe-touch weight bearing for 6 weeks.[1] Patients can then be treated with pool therapy for 4 weeks with progressive weight bearing. Core body strengthening is subsequently accomplished with 8 weeks of land-based physical therapy.

Currently, there are no formal guidelines outlined for ambulation following MIS SIJ fusion; however, known limitations regarding weight-bearing activity between 0 to 6 and 6 to 12 weeks exist, as it takes a minimum of 6 weeks for the fusion to occur. These limitations are often determined on a case-by-case basis and are influenced by patient factors such as osteoporosis and obesity as well as surgical technique. Patients undergoing posterior approach surgical techniques with the use of hardware such as cages are advised to avoid activities that stress the SIJ. Specific limitations include restriction of lifting greater than 10 pounds, limiting bending at the waist, and trying to avoid bearing weight on the operative-side leg for prolonged periods.[2] Patients are typically advised to wear a sacral belt to serve as postoperative bracing for 3 months. Postoperative imaging may be employed, potentially a computed tomography (CT) scan, at the 6-month interval. If no issues are identified, patients may return to full activity.

When the fusion is performed via the lateral approach using triangular titanium implants, they can be placed either "in joint" or "out of joint."[3] When the implants are placed using the "out of joint" technique, the joint stability is at higher risk, leading to stricter limitation on weight-bearing activity. For this approach, it is recommended that ambulatory assist devices such as a walker or cane be used for 6 weeks following surgery. While ambulating, patients are encouraged to use the toe-touch technique to avoid applying any weight on the surgical-side lower extremity.

If the "in joint" technique is performed, joint stability is thought to be more dependable, thus leading to more lenient activity restrictions. It is still recommended that patients use an ambulatory assist device for the first 3 weeks; however, they can apply up to 20 pounds of weight to the operative lower extremity during this time. Following the first 3 weeks of recovery, patients can ambulate without an assist device, as their strength and balance allows. For obese patients, it is recommended that they use a walker or crutches for the entire 6 weeks and avoid bearing more than 20 pounds of weight on the surgical side. These guidelines may have to be adjusted on a patient-by-patient basis, if they have severe osteoporosis or difficulty with balance secondary to other comorbidities like stroke.

Ambulation guidelines are less restrictive for the posterior approach. Following this approach patients are capable of undergoing unassisted ambulation as early as postoperative day 1. They will want to avoid lifting more than 8 pounds as well as bending or twisting at the waist. Patients are permitted to go up and down stairs as tolerated; however, they will want to use handrails to avoid falling, which would be detrimental to their recovery.

Following surgery, patients will also need to perform progressive physical therapy in order to improve muscle strength and increase range of motion. Primary muscle groups that need to heal include the hip extensors and hip abductors (gluteus maximus, gluteus medius, and gluteus minimus). During the first 3 weeks postoperatively, the patient will be working with physical therapy twice a week, taking these muscles through passive range of motion. During this same period it is important to avoid taking the joint through maximum hip flexion and adduction. As tissue healing progresses, so can the amount of resistance that is added in order to improve strength and balance. Prior to surgery the ipsilateral side is most likely weak secondary to pain while the contralateral side is forced to overcompensate, which will result in asymmetry. These muscle groups will need to be retrained in order to improve symmetry, strength, and balance. Increasing resistance allows the patient to lift up to 10 pounds as well as remove restrictions on time spent ambulating.

When considering the posterior approach, the timeline for activity and exercise is much less restrictive. Patients can begin walking immediately if tolerated and can expect to walk as much as a mile within the first month or two. The average return to work was 47 days unless the patient performed heavy labor, which pushed the return date to 2 months. In this respect, too, this varies sharply based on the particular technique. For example, with the percutaneous posterior bone allograft procedure, patients are only restricted from activity that places a high stress on the SIJ. Therefore, these patients can return to work within days of the procedure as long as their occupation is not too physically demanding.

Postoperative infection

Postoperative infection is another area of concern that is monitored in the immediate post-operative period. Martin et al.[4] summarized the Level IV studies on triangular implants, which included a total of 361 patients; only six cases (1.6%) were found to be complicated postoperatively by infection. These findings are similar to those by Shamrock et al.,[5] who summarized a total of 819 SIJ fusions and found that wound infection occurred in 17 (2.0%). Infection accounted for roughly 11% of all complications, the most of any category. According to the North American Spine Society (NASS) data, the occurrence of wound infection in spine surgery despite the administration of appropriate prophylactic antibiotics ranges from 0.7% to 10%.[6]

Prophylactic antibiotic guidelines published by NASS include intravenous administration 30 minutes prior to incision and every 3 hours as needed after uncomplicated spinal surgery. Kakimaru et al.[7] performed a retrospective comparative study comparing surgical site infections in those who received intraoperative prophylactic antibiotics versus those who received intraoperative and postoperative prophylactic antibiotics. Average duration of the postoperative antibiotic course was 2.7 days. A total of 284 patients were reviewed; 143 of them received only intraoperative antibiotics while 141 received intraoperative and postoperative antibiotics. Surgical site infection rate was 1.4% (2/143) and 2.8% (4/141) respectively, indicating that postoperative antibiotic administration does not reduce surgical site infections and is therefore deemed unnecessary.

With MIS techniques, the time to healing is likely shorter and the risk of surgical site infection presumably shorter. Compared to the open surgical techniques, MIS offers a shorter incision length, a shorter duration of operating time, and decreased tissue disruption. It is likely that all of these factors combined result in a lower incidence of surgical site infection in comparison to the open surgical technique.[8,9]

Wound care

Standard wound care guidelines should be followed in the immediate postoperative period. MIS has allowed for a decreased incision size, which reduces the rate of wound complications. Most incisions will be covered with Steri-Strips and possibly staples to help prevent wound dehiscence. It is recommended that patients keep the Steri-Strips on until postoperative day 7 to 10, at which time they can be removed. If staples are present, they can be removed in the office by either the primary care physician or a member of the interventional/surgical team. It is important for the patient to keep the wound dry for the first 48 hours and avoid soaking in a body of water for the first month. Showering is permitted as long as the patient avoids scrubbing directly over the incision. Patients will need to monitor for drainage as well as erythema, swelling, and temperatures greater than 101°F (38.3°C).

Blood loss

Blood loss is minimal in most MIS approaches to the SIJ. Even MIS approaches using hardware, such as a cage, typically have less than 100 mL of estimated blood loss during a surgical case.[2] Blood loss during percutaneous fusion with bone graft is minimal, typically less than 20 mL. Therefore, type and screening or crossmatching is not typically necessary as part of the operative planning. While localized hematomas, ecchymosis, or bruising could potentially occur in frail or thin patients, these can be monitored conservatively and do not typically require any active treatment or intervention.

Postoperative course

The need for and duration of hospitalization following SIJ fusion are directly related to the surgical approach and technique. Patients undergoing an open approach are typically admitted following their procedure. Length of stay can range from 2 to 5 days, with most patients admitted for just over 3 days. Hospitalization and length of stay for the MIS approach vary based on the particular approach. MIS approaches involving significant hardware may require a hospital stay of anywhere from 1 to 4 days, with most patients admitted for about 2 days.

Bone healing and fusion progression should be considered when selecting pain medications postoperatively. Nonsteroidal anti-inflammatory drugs (NSAIDs) are commonly employed for pain control. Ketorolac is often administered for pain control in the postanesthesia care unit (PACU). Ibuprofen, naproxen, meloxicam, and diclofenac are commonly used for subacute pain during the post-discharge course. In patients with gastric comorbidities, COX selective agents are often employed.

In Sivaganesan et al.'s systematic review in 2017, no Level I evidence was found regarding the effect of NSAIDs on fusion rate.[10] Nearly all human studies after 2005 indicate that there is no diminished fusion outcome with NSAID duration of less than 2 weeks. In addition, dose-dependent decreases in fusion rate are not observed when NSAIDs are only used for less than 48 hours after surgery. Patients with chronic use of NSAIDs should be advised to reduce or discontinue NSAIDs in the perioperative period if possible, but NSAID use is not a contraindication.[11] There are some studies that have failed to show clear evidence of fusion impairment with NSAID consumption.[12,13] Given that narcotic use can increase in the absence of NSAIDs, it is possible that a low-dose, limited-duration course of NSAIDs in the postoperative period may be of benefit. While protracted courses of steroids are not advisable, limited single doses such as those used for prophylaxis of postoperative nausea and vomiting should not impact bone healing.

Complications can also vary widely. Although rare, they are most common with open surgical technique or with MIS techniques involving significant hardware. There have been a few reports of pulmonary embolism following surgery.[1] Occasional reports of erosion by the hardware or nerve root irritation are also seen in the literature. There have been no reports of pulmonary embolism following MIS SIJ fusion with percutaneous bone graft. This is intuitive, as postoperative deep venous thrombosis and subsequent pulmonary embolism are likely related to prolonged periods of decreased mobility with more invasive surgical approaches to SIJ fusion.

Pain scores and follow-up

Following MIS SIJ fusion, pain scores and improvements from preoperative scores are some of the primary outcomes discussed when comparing the MIS procedure with open surgical fusion. Many studies have evaluated and compared the results of procedures, stratifying by techniques and approaches. Smith et al.[14] compared the results of open SIJ fusion ($n = 149$) versus MIS SIJ fusion using triangular titanium implants. Twelve months

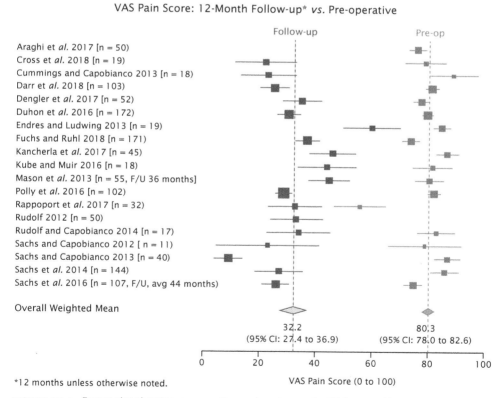

FIGURE 21.1. Forest plot showing preoperative and postoperative VAS scores.[14]

following the procedure, visual analog scale (VAS) pain scores were evaluated for patients in both categories. Pain scores improved by 2.7 points in the open group and 6.2 points in the MIS group. Subsequent follow-up was performed for 96 patients and found that overall scores had improved by 2 points in the open group and 5.6 points in the MIS from preoperative levels.

A study performed by Ledonio et al.[15] compared operations performed at two institutions, including 22 open and 17 MIS SIJ fusions using triangular titanium implant. Oswestry Disability Index (ODI) scores improved from (median) 64 to 46 in the open group and 53 to 13 in the MIS group. The ODI change was larger for the MIS group by a median of 9 points. Fuchs and Ruhl[16] performed a prospective study involving 20 hospitals that included 171 patients who underwent distraction arthrodesis using the DIANA cage. The ODI improved from 51 to 33 and pain as measured by the VAS decreased from 74 to 37 points. Duhon et al.[17] reported 24-month follow-up of a prospective, multi-center single-arm study of 172 patients. In this study, SIJ pain decreased from 79.8 at baseline to 26.0, and ODI decreased from 55.2 at baseline to 30.9 at 24 months. As demonstrated by these studies, pain scores following MIS SIJ fusion have decreased significantly in nearly each study. These findings[4] are concisely demonstrated in Figures 21.1, 21.2, and 21.3.

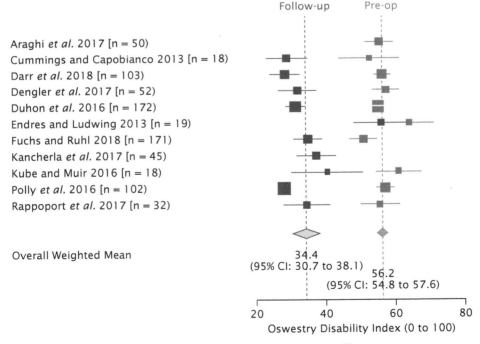

FIGURE 21.2. Forest plot of preoperative and postoperative ODI scores.[14]

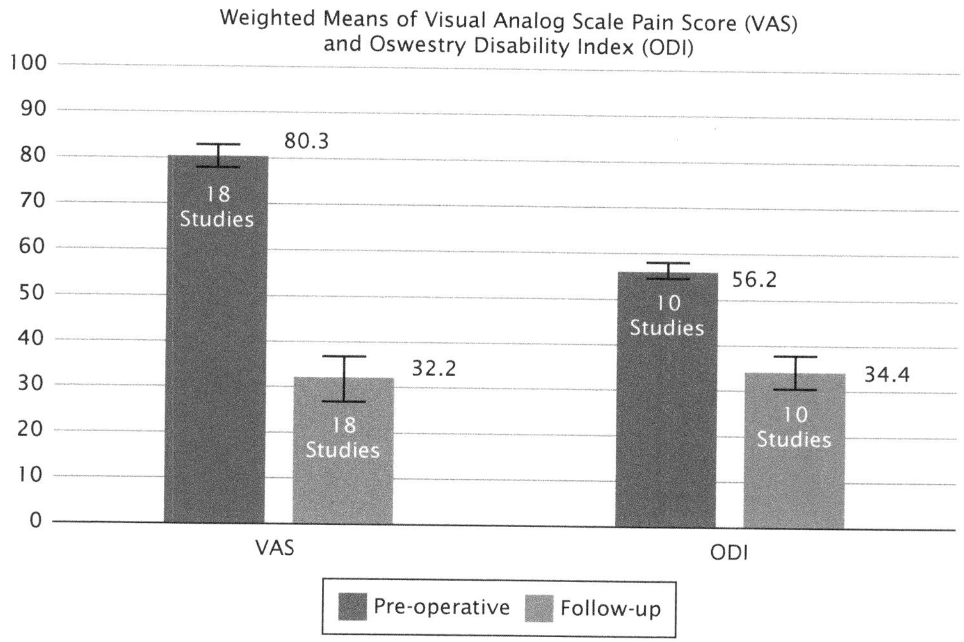

Weighted means calculated by OpenMeta meta-analysis software using the DerSimonian-Laird method in a continuous random effects model. Error bars are 95% confidence intervals.

FIGURE 21.3. Pooled analysis of weighted means for preoperative and postoperative VAS and ODI scores.[14]

References

1. Ledonio CG, Polly DW, Swiontkowski MF. Minimally invasive versus open sacroiliac joint fusion: Are they similarly safe and effective. *Clin Orthop Rel Res.* 2014;472(6):1831–1838.

2. Wise CL, Dall BE. Minimally invasive sacroiliac arthrodesis: Outcomes of a new technique. *J Spinal Disord Tech.* 2008;21(8):579–584.

3. Duhon BS, Cher DJ, Wine KD, et al. Safety and 6-month effectiveness of minimally invasive sacroiliac joint fusion: A prospective study. *Med Devices.* 2013;6:219–229. doi:10.2147/MDER.S55197. PMID: 24363562; PMCID: PMC3865972.

4. Martin CT, Haase L, Lender PA, Polly DW. Minimally invasive sacroiliac joint fusion: The current evidence. *Int J Spine Surg.* 2020;14(Suppl 1):20–29. doi:10.14444/6072

5. Shamrock AG, Patel A, Alam M, Shamrock KH, Al Maaieh M. The Safety Profile of Percutaneous Minimally Invasive Sacroiliac Joint Fusion. *Global Spine Journal* 2019;9(8):874–880.

6. Watters WC, Baisden J, Bono CM, Heggeness MH, Resnick DK, Shaffer WO, Toton JF. Antibiotic prophylaxis in spine surgery: an evidence-based clinical guideline for the use of prophylactic antibiotics in spine surgery. *The Spine Journal: Official Journal of the North American Spine Society* 2009;9(2):142–146.

7. Kakimaru H, Kono M, Matsusaki M, Iwata A, Uchio Y. Postoperative antimicrobial prophylaxis following spinal decompression surgery: is it necessary. *Journal of Orthopaedic Science: Official Journal of the Japanese Orthopaedic Association* 2010;15(3):305–309.

8. Pull ter Gunne AF, Cohen DB. Incidence, prevalence, and analysis of risk factors for surgical site infection following adult spinal surgery. *Spine.* 2009;34(13):1422–1428.

9. Skråmm I, Saltytė Benth J, Bukholm G. Decreasing time trend in SSI incidence for orthopaedic procedures: Surveillance matters. *J Hosp Infect.* 2012;82(4):243–247.

10. Sivaganesan A, Chotai S, White-Dzuro G, et al. The effect of NSAIDs on spinal fusion: A cross-disciplinary review of biochemical, animal, and human studies. *Eur Spine J*. 2017;26:2719–2728.

11. Thaller J, Walker M, Kline AJ, Anderson DG. The effect of nonsteroidal anti-inflammatory agents on spinal fusion. *Orthopedics*. 2005;28:299–305.

12. Marquez-Lara A, Hutchinson ID, Nuñez F, et al. Nonsteroidal anti-inflammatory drugs and bone healing: A systematic review of research quality. *J Bone Joint Surg Rev*. 2016;4(3);01874474-201603000-00005.

13. Lisowska B, Kosson D, Domaracka K. Positives and negatives of nonsteroidal anti-inflammatory drugs in bone healing: The effects of these drugs on bone repair. *Drug Des Devel Ther*. 2018;12:1809–1814.

14. Smith AG, Capobianco R, Cher D, et al. Open versus minimally invasive sacroiliac joint fusion: A multi-center comparison of perioperative measures and clinical outcomes. *Ann Surg Innov Res*. 2013;7(1):14.

15. Ledonio CG, Polly DW, Jr, Swiontkowski MF, Cummings JT, Jr. Comparative effectiveness of open versus minimally invasive sacroiliac joint fusion. *Med Devices*. 2014;7:187–193.

16. Fuchs V, Ruhl B. Distraction arthrodesis of the sacroiliac joint: 2-year results of a descriptive prospective multi-center cohort study in 171 patients. *Eur Spine J*. 2018;27(1):194–204.

17. Duhon BS, Bitan F, Lockstadt H, et al. Triangular titanium implants for minimally invasive sacroiliac joint fusion: 2-year follow-up from a prospective multicenter trial. *Int J Spine Surg*. 2016;10:13.

22

Complications and their management

Hemant Kalia

Introduction

Minimally invasive (MIS) sacroiliac joint (SIJ) fusion is becoming increasingly popular for treatment of chronic pain attributable to SIJ etiology. The incidence rate of chronic low back pain secondary to SIJ pathology ranges between 15% and 30%.[1] Due to overlapping referral patterns from lumbar internal disc disruption, facet joint arthritis, SIJ etiology, and post-laminectomy fusion construct, the true prevalence rates of low back and buttock pain attributable specifically to SIJ pathology are hard to determine.[2,3]

Historically, SIJ arthrodesis has been commonly performed through an open surgical approach in cases of recalcitrant pain attributable to SIJ pathology.[4] However, the open approach carries significant risk associated with surgical site infection, long incisions, extended hospital stay, bone harvesting, and neurologic injury.[5] The MIS approach to joint fusion was first reported in 2004 with the goal of decreasing the complications associated with open surgical fusions.[4,6,7]

Since the advent of MIS SIJ fusion surgery, several studies have confirmed its clinical efficacy in treating SIJ pain, specifically with low rates of adverse events and reoperation as compared with open surgery. Most of these studies have focused on efficacy and patient satisfaction; very few studies have focused on the safety of the procedure, and even in those, their small sample sizes could not provide any statistically significant conclusions.[6,8–10]

Surgical complications and management

The current MIS approach to SIJ fusion is safe and effective. Most of the studies included the lateral approach using titanium rods. The overall complication rates of MIS lateral SIJ fusion ranges between 3.5% and 18%.[6,11,12] Miller et al. reported an overall complication rate of 3.5% to 5.6%; this is the lowest reported in the literature, but their study was industry sponsored and required spontaneous reporting, thereby creating a bias.[11]

Some of the common complications reported during and after MIS SIJ fusion are infections and neurovascular injuries. Over the past few years, multiple techniques have gained popularity, focusing on the posterior approach to percutaneously fuse the SIJ. As there is no major neurovascular bundle anatomically located along the posterior aspect of the SIJ, theoretically this approach should be even safer than the lateral approach. There are no long-term prospective studies elucidating the safety or efficacy of the posterior approach in the literature at this time. There are a few case reports and case series that establish the merit of this approach, but well-designed prospective studies are required to confirm the veracity of these initial clinical trends.

Infection

Preoperative prevention

Patients with active infections are not candidates for SIJ fusion. In questionable situations, obtaining a complete blood count with differential analysis, urinalysis, and erythrocyte sedimentation rate can help identify at-risk patients. Depending on the location and severity of an earlier bacterial infection, implant surgery may be postponed until an antibiotic course is completed and symptoms and laboratory studies have returned to normal. We strongly suggest following the best practices for preventing surgical site infections. The infection control strategy for the posterior approach to SIJ fusion should be similar to any other advanced interventional spine and pain procedure. The Neurostimulation Appropriateness Consensus Committee (NACC)'s recommendations for infection prevention and management can also be considered in the interim until there are specific guidelines related to SIJ fusion using the posterior approach.[13]

Postoperative infection

Surgical site infection is the bane of any surgical procedure. Schoell et al.[12] reported an infection rate of 4.1% within 6 months of MIS SIJ fusion; the infection rate was 2.9% in the first 6 months and increased to 4.9% at 12 months. A systematic review of similar procedures like minimally invasive spine discectomy, foraminotomy, decompression, and fusion reported an infection rate of 1.1%.[14] Although there is a striking difference between the technique and approach of these procedures and SIJ fusion, the lateral approach using titanium rods has been associated with higher rates of infection as compared with these similar spinal implant procedures.

Interestingly, urinary tract infections are also quite common after the lateral approach of SIJ fusion. One study reported an infection rate of 3.8% at 90 days and 4.9% at 6 months, with infection being more common in females than males.[12]

Neurovascular injuries

Preoperative prevention

The only weapon with which the unconscious patient can immediately retaliate upon the incompetent surgeon is hemorrhage.
William S. Halsted

Vascular complications related to patient-specific risk factors can be prevented with astute preoperative planning and care. One of the common reasons for bleeding or hematoma formation is the underlying use of anticoagulation and antiplatelet agents. The authors recommend following the published guidelines titled "Interventional Spine and Pain Procedures in Patients on Antiplatelet and Anticoagulant Medications (Second Edition)," which are widely used in the practice of interventional pain and are endorsed by most of the societies (American Society of Regional Anesthesia and Pain Medicine, the European Society of Regional Anesthesia and Pain Therapy, the American Academy of Pain Medicine, the International Neuromodulation Society, the North American Neuromodulation Society, and the World Institute of Pain).[15] We would suggest categorizing MIS SIJ fusion using the posterior approach as a high-risk procedure as per the ASRA guidelines.

Postoperative hematoma and neural injury

The MIS approach to SIJ fusion is associated with fewer complications than the open approach. In one of the studies comparing the open versus the MIS approach, the authors were able to show that patients in the open group had increased blood loss and a longer mean surgical time and length of stay than those undergoing the minimally invasive approach.[1]

Percutaneous SIJ fusion using the lateral approach with titanium rods has been associated with a significant risk of neurovascular injury, primarily due to the anatomic location of the neurovascular bundle along the lateral border of the sacrum. The incidence rate of neural injury is about 4.3% in the first 90 days and 6.2% at 6 months.[12]

References

1. Ledonio CGT, Polly DW, Swiontkowski MF. Minimally invasive versus open sacroiliac joint fusion: Are they similarly safe and effective? Clin Orthop Rel Res 2014;472:1831–1838.
2. DePalma MJ, Ketchum JM, Saullo TR. Etiology of chronic low back pain in patients having undergone lumbar fusion. Pain Med 2011;12(5):732–739.
3. Depalma MJ, Ketchum JM, Trussell BS, et al. Does the location of low back pain predict its source? PM R 2011;3(1):33–39.
4. Lorio MP, Polly Jr. DW, Ninkovic I, et al. Utilization of minimally invasive surgical approach for sacroiliac joint fusion in surgeon population of ISASS and SMISS membership. Open Orthop J 2014;8(1):1–6.
5. Al-Khayer A, Hegarty J, Hahn D, Grevitt MP. Percutaneous sacroiliac joint arthrodesis: A novel technique. J Spinal Disord Tech. 2008;21(5):359–363.
6. Smith AG, Capobianco R, Cher D, et al. Open versus minimally invasive sacroiliac joint fusion: A multi-center comparison of perioperative measures and clinical outcomes. Ann Surg Innov Res 2013;7(1):1–12.
7. Rudolf L. Sacroiliac joint arthrodesis: MIS technique with titanium implants: Report of the first 50 patients and outcomes. Open Orthop J 2012;6(1):495–502.
8. Sachs D, Capobianco R. Minimally invasive sacroiliac joint fusion: One-year outcomes in 40 patients. Adv Orthop 2013;2013:1–5.
9. Cummings J, Capobianco RA. Minimally invasive sacroiliac joint fusion: One-year outcomes in 18 patients. Ann Surg Innov Res 2013;7(1):1–7.
10. Duhon B, Cher D, Wine K, et al. Safety and 6-month effectiveness of minimally invasive sacroiliac joint fusion: A prospective study. Med Devices 2013;6:219–229.

11. Miller LE, Carlton Reckling W, Block JE. Analysis of postmarket complaints database for the iFuse SI joint fusion system®: A minimally invasive treatment for degenerative sacroiliitis and sacroiliac joint disruption. Med Devices Evid Res 2013;6(1):77–84.

12. Schoell K, Buser Z, Jakoi A, et al. Postoperative complications in patients undergoing minimally invasive sacroiliac fusion. Spine J 2016;16(11):1324–1332.

13. Deer TR, Provenzano DA, Hanes M, et al. The Neurostimulation Appropriateness Consensus Committee (NACC) recommendations for infection prevention and management. Neuromodulation 2017;20(1):31–50.

14. Kane J, Kay A, Maltenfort M, Kepler C, et al. Complication rates of minimally invasive spine surgery compared to open surgery: A systematic literature review. Sem Spine Surg 2013;25(3):191–199.

15. Narouze S, Benzon HT, Provenzano D, et al. Interventional spine and pain procedures in patients on antiplatelet and anticoagulant medications (second edition): Guidelines from the American Society of Regional Anesthesia and Pain Medicine, the European Society of Regional Anaesthesia and Pain Therapy, the American Academy of Pain Medicine, the International Neuromodulation Society, the North American Neuromodulation Society, and the World Institute of Pain. Reg Anesth Pain Med 2018;43(3).

23

What if fusion fails?

Hemant Kalia

Introduction

Lumbar degenerative disc disease, lumbar facet arthropathy, and sacroiliac joint (SIJ) pathologies are the top three etiologies of chronic low back pain. The SIJ plays a role in 15% to 30% cases of chronic low back pain,[1–3] and it is even more common (40%) in patients with a history of prior lumbar fusion, primarily due to adjacent-level disease.[4] Treatments for SIJ disease include physical therapy, nonsteroidal anti-inflammatory medications, complementary medical approaches, intraarticular steroid injections, radiofrequency ablation (RFA), and both open and minimally invasive (MIS) lateral and posterior joint fixation and fusion.[5–8]

There are several implants and approaches available for SIJ fusion or fixation. The strategy can include fixation only or fixation and fusion.

Fixation strategies include the placement of different types of screws or plates across the joint line posteriorly to fixate the joint. The SIJ is a complex C-shaped or L-shaped joint that requires more in-depth biomechanical analyses in order to better predict the risk of failure or instability of the joint after fixation.[9]

Fusion strategies range from joint disruption and implantation of allograft to implantation of devices with special coatings that promote bony ingrowth. SIJ fusion and fixation both lead to stabilization of the SIJ, whereas SIJ fusion leads to transfixation across the joint line with bony ingrowth leading to long-term immobility.[10]

What if the fusion fails? This question is important to patients and their surgeons and interventionalists alike. To answer this question, it is important to understand the basics of fusion and fixation physiology. There are several risk factors, which can be broadly classified as either patient-related or device/approach-related factors that predispose to surgical failure. Timely identification and appropriate management of these risk factors can improve outcomes.

Risk factors for fusion failure

The risk of fusion failure can be minimized by (1) optimizing medical comorbidities, (2) eliminating the risk factors that can interfere with bone healing, and (3) using surgical techniques that promote bone growth to achieve solid fusion. The risk factors for fusion failure can be broadly classified into two categories: those related to the patient (smoking, age-related osteoporosis, rheumatoid arthritis, diabetes mellitus, hyperparathyroidism, poor nutritional status, systemic inflammatory diseases) and those related to the device or approach. The underlying physiologic, biologic, and molecular events crucial to the process of fusion are poorly understood. Moreover, lack of predictive noninvasive techniques for evaluating arthrodesis further limits clinical studies.[11,12]

Comprehensive knowledge of different categories of bone graft substitutes and the biology of healing in different types of fusion and fixation approaches can help interventionalists improve their surgical outcomes. Osteoconductive (collagen, ceramics, polymers, and corals) and osteoinductive (BMP, PDGF, TGF-b, VEGF) substitutes can play a vital role in successful fusion.

Adhering to the basic principles of spinal fusion surgery, coupled with systematic identification and targeting of factors that led to the previous fusion failure, will increase the likelihood of a successful revision fusion.[11]

Posterior approach

Allograft

SIJ fusion via the posterior approach is most commonly being done using allografts. These allografts, although safe and effective, can be a challenge if deployed incorrectly. Once deployed between the lateral and medial joint surface, their retrieval using the percutaneous approach can be cumbersome and risky. Special attention should be paid to the point of fixation. There is also a dearth of literature regarding the long-term efficacy and extent of fusion based on the number of allografts used.

Screws and plates

Transarticular screws and plates have been used to successfully fuse the SIJ, but the long-term efficacy and durability of this approach still need to be studied and reported in the literature. If deployed incorrectly, screws and plates can be easily retrieved via an open approach.

Lateral approach

The triangular implant system is designed to be deployed using a lateral approach to fuse the SIJ. Most of these procedures are done by spine surgeons under general anesthesia and carry significant risk for neurovascular bundle injury with protracted recovery.[9] If deployed incorrectly, retrieval of this system can lead to considerable morbidity due to the anatomic location of this system.

Neuroablation

SIJ-mediated pain recalcitrant to conservative and advanced treatment options, including SIJ fusion, can benefit from thermal RFA of the L5 primary dorsal ramus and sacral dorsal rami lateral branches at S1, S2, and S3. There is a growing body of evidence supporting the efficacy of radiofrequency neurotomy for SIJ posterior ligament complex pain.[13-16] Patel et al. reported successful treatment of SIJ pain with cooled RFA in 59% of their patients at the end of 9 months.[17]

Neuromodulation

Pain transduction can be successfully modulated by targeting peripheral nerves, spinal cord, and spinal cord radices to cause pain relief.[18] Patients who fail to respond to conservative treatment options or have failed SIJ fusion can be considered for advanced neuromodulation treatment options. Guentchev et al. published their 12-month experience using peripheral nerve stimulation in patients with chronic low back pain attributable to SIJ pathology. In their case series, they reported reduction of the visual analog scale (VAS) score from 8 to 1.7, with preoperative pain medication reduction by at least 50%.[19] In another case report, Kim et al. successfully implanted a quad lead along the left S1 nerve root using a cephalocaudal approach at the L4–5 interlaminar epidural space to target SIJ-mediated left buttock pain.[20] S3 nerve root neuroaugmentation was reported to be a viable option in providing adequate pain relief in two patients with severe SIJ pain unresponsive to conventional therapy.[21] Sacral neuromodulation can also be considered in cases of intractable SIJ-mediated pain.[20]

Conclusion

MIS SIJ fixation and fusion are effective treatment options for identified SIJ pathology. Surgical revision is more commonly seen after SIJ fixation using screws as compared to SIJ fusion.[10] Patient-related risk factors for development of pseudoarthrosis should be appropriately identified and addressed in a timely manner. The device and surgical approach may make an important difference in the overall success of MIS SIJ fusion.

References

1. Maigne J-Y, Aivaliklis A, Pfefer F. Results of sacroiliac joint double block and value of sacroiliac pain provocation tests in 54 patients with low back pain. Spine 1996;21(16):1889–1892.
2. DePalma MJ, Ketchum JM, Saullo TR. Etiology of chronic low back pain in patients having undergone lumbar fusion. Pain Med 2011;12(5):732–739.
3. DePalma MJ, Ketchum JM, Saullo T. What is the source of chronic low back pain and does age play a role? Pain Med 2011;12(2):224–233.
4. Liliang PC, Lu K, Liang CL, et al. Sacroiliac joint pain after lumbar and lumbosacral fusion: Findings using dual sacroiliac joint blocks. Pain Med 2011;12(4):565–570.
5. Slipman CW, Lipetz JS, Plastaras CT, et al. Fluoroscopically guided therapeutic sacroiliac joint injections for sacroiliac joint syndrome. Am J Phys Med Rehabil 2001;80(6):425–432.

6. Cohen SP. Sacroiliac joint pain: A comprehensive review of anatomy, diagnosis, and treatment. Anesth Analg 2005;101(5):1440–1453.

7. Sachs D, Capobianco R. Minimally invasive sacroiliac joint fusion: One-year outcomes in 40 patients. Adv Orthop 2013;2013:1–5.

8. Smith AG, Capobianco R, Cher D, et al. Open versus minimally invasive sacroiliac joint fusion: A multi-center comparison of perioperative measures and clinical outcomes. Ann Surg Innov Res 2013;7(1):1–12.

9. Casaroli G, Bassani T, Brayda-Bruno M, et al. What do we know about the biomechanics of the sacro-iliac joint and of sacropelvic fixation? A literature review. Med Eng Phys 2020;76:1–12.

10. Spain K, Holt T. Surgical revision after sacroiliac joint fixation or fusion. Int J Spine Surg 2017;11(1):24–30.

11. Boden SD. Overview of the biology of lumbar spine fusion and principles for selecting a bone graft substitute Spine 2002;27(16 Suppl 1):S26–S31.

12. Brodsky AE, Kovalsky ES, Khalil MA. Correlation of radiologic assessment of lumbar spine fusions with surgical exploration. Spine 1991;16(6S):S261–S265.

13. Patel N. Twelve-month follow-up of a randomized trial assessing cooled radiofrequency denervation as a treatment for sacroiliac region pain. Pain Pract 2016;16(2):154–167.

14. Davis T, Loudermilk E, DePalma M, et al. Prospective, multicenter, randomized, crossover clinical trial comparing the safety and effectiveness of cooled radiofrequency ablation with corticosteroid injection in the management of knee pain from osteoarthritis. Reg Anesth Pain Med 2018;43(1):84–91.

15. Deer TR, Esposito MF, McRoberts WP, et al. A systematic literature review of peripheral nerve stimulation therapies for the treatment of pain. Pain Med 2020;21(8):1590–603.

16. Yang AJ, McCormick ZL, Zheng PZ, Schneider BJ. Radiofrequency ablation for posterior sacroiliac joint complex pain: A narrative review. PM R 2019;11:S105–S113.

17. Patel N, Gross A, Brown L, Gekht G. A randomized, placebo-controlled study to assess the efficacy of lateral branch neurotomy for chronic sacroiliac joint pain. Pain Med 2012;13(3):383–398.

18. Deer TR, Naidu R, Strand N, et al. A review of the bioelectronic implications of stimulation of the peripheral nervous system for chronic pain conditions. Bioelectron Med 2020;6:9.

19. Guentchev M, Preuss C, Rink R, et al. Technical note: Treatment of sacroiliac joint pain with peripheral nerve stimulation. Neuromodulation 2015;18(5):392–396.

20. Kim YH, Moon DE. Sacral nerve stimulation for the treatment of sacroiliac joint dysfunction: A case report. Neuromodulation 2010;13(4):306–310.

21. Calvillo O, Esses SI, Ponder C, et al. Neuroaugmentation in the management of sacroiliac joint pain: Report of two cases. Spine 1998;23(9):1069–1072.

Index

Tables, figures and boxes are indicated by *t*, *f* and *b* following the page number